INTERMITTENT FASTING SOLUTIONS FOR WOMEN OVER 50

ELEVATE MOOD AND ENERGY, IMPROVE YOUR HEALTH, UNDERSTAND HORMONES, SHED WEIGHT, AND EMBRACE AGING WITH CONFIDENCE

MAXINE MORRIS STEWART

© **Copyright 2024 - All rights reserved.**

The content contained within this book may not be reproduced, duplicated or transmitted without direct written permission from the author or the publisher.

Under no circumstances will any blame or legal responsibility be held against the publisher, or author, for any damages, reparation, or monetary loss due to the information contained within this book, either directly or indirectly.

Legal Notice:

This book is copyright protected. It is only for personal use. You cannot amend, distribute, sell, use, quote or paraphrase any part, or the content within this book, without the consent of the author or publisher.

Disclaimer Notice:

Please note the information contained within this document is for educational and entertainment purposes only. All effort has been executed to present accurate, up to date, reliable, complete information. No warranties of any kind are declared or implied. Readers acknowledge that the author is not engaged in the rendering of legal, financial, medical or professional advice. The content within this book has been derived from various sources. Please consult a licensed professional before attempting any techniques outlined in this book.

By reading this document, the reader agrees that under no circumstances is the author responsible for any losses, direct or indirect, that are incurred as a result of the use of the information contained within this document, including, but not limited to, errors, omissions, or inaccuracies.

TABLE OF CONTENTS

Introduction   5

1. THE FASCINATING HISTORY OF FASTING   9
   What's Intermittent Fasting All About?   10
   The Science of Intermittent Fasting   17
2. PREPARING TO FAST   23
   Common Misperceptions About Fasting   24
   Pre-Fasting Evaluation   25
   Tips For Mentally Preparing For The Fasting Journey: 28
   Building a Strong Foundation   31
3. FIND THE BEST METHOD FOR YOU   37
   Time-Restricted Eating   38
   The 5:2 Diet and Variations   42
4. UNLOCK THE POWER OF BALANCED NUTRITION   47
   Nutrition Basics   48
   Designing Nutrient-Dense Meals   51
   Hydration and Intermittent Fasting   62
5. BREAK THROUGH BARRIERS, PLATEAUS, AND OBSTACLES   65
   Dealing With Hunger and Cravings   66
   Plateaus and Progress Stalls   74
6. UNDERSTAND THE IMPACT OF MENOPAUSE ON HORMONES   81
   Hormonal Changes in Women Over 50   81
   Menopause and the Risk of Osteoporosis   86
   Assessing and Reducing Fracture Risk   87
   Hormone Replacement Therapy (HRT)   90
   Safeguard Your Health   92
   Navigating Menopause With Intermittent Fasting   93

7. HOW FASTING AND EXERCISE WORK
   TOGETHER   97
   The Synergy of Exercise and Fasting   98
   Fasting and Muscle Preservation   116

8. NOURISH YOUR MIND   119
   The Impact of Fasting on Brain Function   121
   Fasting Versus Neurodegenerative Diseases   124
   Nutrients for Cognitive Health   126

9. STRENGTHEN YOUR HEART   133
   Understanding Heart Health In Women Over 50   134
   Heart-Healthy Nutrition and Fasting   139

10. LONG-TERM BENEFITS EQUALS SUCCESS   145
    Intermittent Fasting, Healthy Aging, and Longevity 146
    Creating a Sustainable Fasting Routine   152

Conclusion   157
Frequently Asked Questions   159
References   167

INTRODUCTION

Seven years ago, I was experiencing extreme abdominal pain and severe overload anxiety. While working full-time and doing clinical rotations for my master's course, I navigated single motherhood with a teen and a tween! Though I was following a healthy diet and swimming three or four times weekly for exercise, my symptoms were wearing me down.

After a thorough medical work-up that included blood tests, breath tests, an endoscopy, and a colonoscopy, I was diagnosed with an irritable bowel syndrome (IBS) flare, lactose intolerance, and small intestinal bacterial overgrowth (SIBO). The best available treatment at the time was a medication costing $1,400 per month—are you kidding me? I politely declined and began a quest for an affordable and effective solution.

I trialed supplements, vitamins, and elimination diets with little to no success. My last ditch effort was intermittent fasting. I'm so thankful I found mention of it in a medical journal and dared to give it a try.

Interestingly, the crippling abdominal pain and cramping from IBS and SIBO went from a daily occurrence to less than a monthly issue almost immediately. That was pretty awesome, given that I didn't change my eating. All I did was fast for at least 14 hours a day.

The benefits haven't waned since I started this practice. However, I've noticed improvements in other areas of my health since becoming more intentional about when and what I eat.

Let's face it: Life brings a lot of unexpected and unwanted changes when you're north of 50.

Some things start to droop south and jiggle east and west. Others begin to bulge along an unseen axis and make unexpected noises at the most inopportune times. Brain fog becomes a constant challenge for some of us, whereas others begin to feel as though the battle to prevent chronic disease is all uphill.

However, we don't have to stay victims to the physiological changes and gravitational pull that often characterize life after 50.

Let me explain.

Though I didn't start it to lose weight, I shed 18 pounds last year in eight months and got my curves back by intermittent fasting the right way. I cut out cheat days with soda and junk food and consistently followed a healthy diet.

While an average of two pounds per month may not seem like much to celebrate, I accomplished this weight loss despite taking a couple week-long trips in six of those eight months. I stayed with family and at resorts and hotels, and never missed an opportunity to have dessert! I wasn't starving myself, but my daily intake was not optimal either.

The unanticipated benefits of intermittent fasting intrigued me so much that I delved deeper into the research and science behind the practice. I discovered many interesting, evidence-based facts, a few stretches of the truth, and several false claims.

The mixed messages in the research increased my desire to dig even more, so I did. After reading countless studies, articles, and books about the subject, I was compelled to write about what I'd learned.

My goal is to show women over 50 how to successfully adopt a lifestyle of intermittent fasting to manage weight, look great, and feel their best while reducing risk factors for chronic disease. I can't wait to guide you on this journey!

This book is best suited for women confused and intimidated about intermittent fasting and a bit afraid to get started. It's also for the countless women who have tried intermittent fasting and failed.

Don't give up just yet!

After reading this book, you'll feel confident and ready to tackle your health and weight goals with intermittent fasting. I want you to have more pep in your step and mental stamina than you ever dreamed of without reinventing the wheel or going through all the legwork I invested in this book.

If you're ready to put an end to fad starvation diets and restrictive eating regimens, look no further. If you're tired of wasting money on diet supplements and medications, gym memberships, or surgery only to see the weight return months later, this book is for you.

In the following chapters, you'll understand how to lose weight with fasting and be even more successful by combining it with nutrient-dense meals and exercise. You'll find seven delicious recipes that can form the basis of your meals, and I'm sure you'll enjoy them. I've also included 12 safe and easy exercises for beginners that are adaptable to intensify a workout.

Here's what's important right now: As you read this book, you'll find answers to questions that will impact your success with intermittent fasting, such as:

- Why does food and drink intake need to change immediately?
- What's the best fasting interval?
- Who should consider intermittent fasting, and who should not?
- What's the best way to get back on track when things don't go as planned?
- What steps are needed to sustain weight and health gains for life?

What are you waiting for? It's time to dig in!

THE FASCINATING HISTORY OF FASTING

I used to think that fasting was just something people did to purge their souls and get closer to God, but boy, was I wrong! Going without food for more than half a day has more physical and mental health benefits than I imagined.

Fasting has been a fundamental part of life for thousands of years, primarily out of necessity. When there was no food to eat, people went hungry for as long as it took until the next opportunity to find and procure a meal, which could be hours or days later.

Over time, people started recognizing patterns and seasonal trends and learned to read the signs of oncoming drought or famine. Learning gave way to planning, preparation, and storing of food. In times of plenty and food security, fasting wasn't on anyone's mind except as it related to spiritual practices.

We have only recently begun to explore and discover the many benefits of fasting that extend beyond weight management and spiritual enlightenment. Now, there are as many different fasts as there are reasons to fast.

I've been intermittent fasting for over seven years; it's the only intervention that consistently manages the IBS that has plagued me since college. Thanks to fasting, my physical and mental health and weight are better now than two decades ago.

WHAT'S INTERMITTENT FASTING ALL ABOUT?

With this type of fasting, you alternate between periods of eating and not eating. Specifically, there are small windows of time during which you consume all of your calories for the day, followed by long periods without caloric intake. Ideally, intermittent fasting regimens last for weeks or months, if not indefinitely.

Before we get too far ahead, let's clarify that intermittent fasting has nothing to do with starving yourself. It's a simple way of giving your gut time to fully process your nutrient intake while creating an opportunity for you to cut down on the calories you consume.

As you fast, your body will burn through readily available carbohydrates first, then turn to fat stores to fuel ongoing physiological processes.

The result is that the fat surrounding your organs and in various areas of your body will be used for fuel through ketosis instead of accumulating. This fat-burning process improves overall health and well-being and leads to weight loss and a trimmer physique for those who do it consistently and well.

Intermittent Fasting Versus Traditional Diets

Both intermittent fasting and traditional diets limit your calories, leading to remarkable weight loss and other health-related benefits—if done correctly. However, strict diets based on counting calories and avoiding certain foods can be challenging to maintain in the long run. Also, foods acceptable with intermittent fasting may not be allowed on a traditional diet.

If you want a sustainable strategy that lets you reap and keep the benefits long-term, intermittent fasting could be the best option. Seven years of traditional dieting is not a realistic weight loss plan, but shedding pounds was a breeze with my fasting regimen. If I can do this, so can you!

Variations of Intermittent Fasting

The wide variety of fasting options makes it easier to choose the type that works for you based on your schedule, job, health, diet, and other vital factors. Let me briefly explain the different versions of intermittent fasting that I came across.

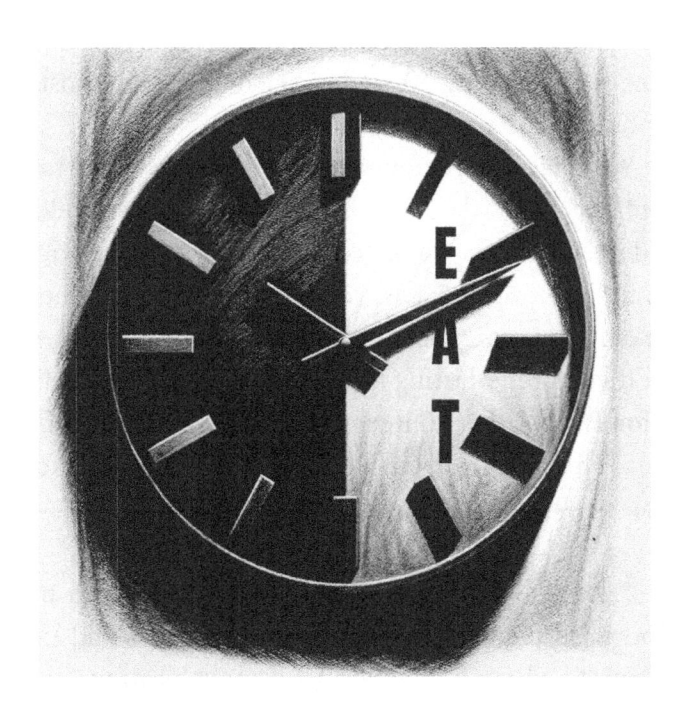

Time-Restricted Eating

This type of fasting, abbreviated as TRE, involves separating your day into periods of eating and fasting. It's one of the most popular methods because you naturally fast when you sleep. The longer you sleep, the longer you can stretch that fasting time.

TRE is a great option for first-timers. Let's look at some standard TRE versions:

- **12:12:** Here, the fasting and eating durations are the same at 12 hours each. This regimen is an excellent option for a first-timer. However, your body starts to burn fat for fuel after about 12 hours of fasting. Moving on to a longer fasting interval as soon as possible is the best way to maximize results.
- **14:10:** You'll fast for 14 hours and consume your calories during the remaining 10, such as 9 a.m. to 7 p.m. Most of your fast will occur while you sleep.
- **16:8:** You'll fast for 16 hours and limit caloric intake to eight hours of the day. For example, your eating window could stretch from 10 a.m. to 6 p.m. If you're in bed by 9 p.m. and wake up at 5 a.m., you'll have fasted for 11 hours, with only five more to go.
- **18:6:** If you prefer fasting for extended periods, the 18:6 version is ideal, though it may be too challenging for first-timers. The prolonged fasting hours can be draining for people not accustomed to going without food.

Beginners, people who have to take medications with meals, or those who have physical jobs will find the 14:10 and the 12:12 versions easy to adopt. Both give a long enough eating window for three to four meals, with plenty of time for digestion.

To ease into fasting, it helps to eat the first meal at the start of the day, followed by lunch about four to five hours later. Time the last meal between three and four hours before bed so you can burn off the calories prior to retiring for the night.

After one to two weeks, keep the same meal times but reduce the caloric intake or portion sizes for each meal. You should be ready to drop one of the meals in a couple more weeks to fast 16 to 18 hours; doing so will maximize fat burning.

If you have to take medications with food three times daily, you may find it impossible to have more than a 14-hour fasting window. Talk to your healthcare provider to see if there's any flexibility in your medication dosing schedule to allow for a more extended fasting period.

Engaging in longer fasting regimens when you're not ready can increase your chances of failure and giving up. Be easy on yourself and take fasting one step at a time.

Whether you start fasting only one, two, or three days per week, consider your overall health goals and stick to your plan. Choose an achievable fasting interval and maintain it for at least four to six weeks to give your body time to adapt.

If you don't see any signs of improvement in weight loss, clothes fitting looser, or increased energy and stamina, expand your fasting to most days of the week. Alternatively, prolong the fasting hours to get closer to the 18:6 version.

Another option to maximize results is to combine the previous methods of intensifying a fast. This strategy will have you fasting on an 18:6 schedule most days of the week.

The 5:2 Method

This "twice-a-week" strategy dictates time and calories. The fasting window is two days, during which you severely limit your total caloric intake to 500 calories over two meals. You eat as usual during the rest of the weekdays.

There's no dietary restriction on foods and drinks with the 5:2 diet, but I recommend those high in nutrients and low in calories. Such options make you feel satiated quickly and for longer, too. Also, the two days of fasting don't have to be consecutive. In fact, make sure there is at least one non-fasting day between them.

The 24-Hour Fast

Some call this the "eat-stop-eat" strategy because you fast for a whole day and eat at your usual time the next day. Whether you prefer to fast from breakfast to breakfast, lunch to lunch, or dinner to dinner, your next meal is always 24 hours away.

The Alternate-Day Fast (ADF)

In this version of intermittent fasting, you eat and drink whatever you want on non-fasting days and don't consume any calories every other day. If you eat from 7 a.m. to 7 p.m. on Monday, you would fast from 7 p.m. to midnight and all of Tuesday. Your next meal would be Wednesday around 7 a.m., for a total fast time of 36 hours.

However, due to dehydration and muscle wasting risks, I wouldn't recommend the ADF as a long-term weight loss strategy. Still, you can reduce risks and maintain benefits from this fast by transitioning to one of the more popular time-restricted regimens mentioned previously.

Other intermittent fasts exist, including "one meal a day" (OMAD) and fasts lasting from 42 to 72 hours or longer. Research on intermittent fasting is ever-changing, with each version offering benefits and varying levels of risk.

Most of the findings and benefits of the longer fasts come from animal studies at this time. Results from human studies have been inconsistent at best and sometimes conflicting.

The TRE methods and the 5:2 fast have been proven safe and effective in research studies, so we'll focus on those. The ADF, OMAD, and longer intermittent fasts are beyond the scope of this book.

Potential Benefits for Women Over 50

Now, let's briefly examine what you stand to gain from intermittent fasting.

- **Weight management:** Many of us become more sedentary as we age, contributing to weight gain. Further, as we pass that 50-year mark, we tend to store fat more and burn it less. If you stick to your fasting plan, you can lose weight and keep it off while getting your curves back, just like I did!
- **Blood sugar regulation:** When the body responds appropriately to insulin, it takes sugar out of the bloodstream. This process is not as efficient in postmenopausal women. Kubala's 2023 study found women over 55 had an improvement in blood sugar levels after just six weeks of following a 16:8 fasting regimen.
- **Enhanced longevity:** Did you know human growth hormone (HGH) levels lower as you age? HGH is involved in metabolism, insulin regulation, and body composition; these factors impact the length of your life. With

intermittent fasting, HGH levels rise, promoting better insulin sensitivity and enhancing longevity
- **Reduced risk of heart disease:** The rate of cardiovascular diseases in women over 50 seems to climb higher every year and is associated with increased levels of bad cholesterol. Fasting lowers bad cholesterol levels.

Who Should Avoid Intermittent Fasting?

While intermittent fasting has a lot of benefits, there are many things to consider before trying it. This type of fasting may prove difficult or may not be for you if any of the following apply:

- **You have sleep issues:** Quality sleep is essential for rejuvenation and healing. If you have insomnia, apnea, or other chronic sleep disorders, first take steps to address them. Hunger related to intermittent fasting can aggravate an existing sleep problem.
- **You have diabetes:** Fasting could be detrimental if you have diabetes and your condition is far from being controlled or if you take insulin. The combination of fasting and medication can cause sugar levels to drop dangerously low and cause you to go into a coma.
- **Your medication requires food:** If you have to take medications with food, intermittent fasting for 16 to 18 hours or more may not be a good option. However, a 14:10 or 12:12 version of fasting may allow you to stick to your medication dosing schedule. Don't change your prescription dosing times on your own without input from your healthcare provider.
- **You have a major illness:** Cancer, eating disorders, and other chronic conditions can greatly compromise your immune system. Your body needs calories to keep your

defense mechanisms active and fight infections and diseases. Intermittent fasting could potentially impair the body's healing capacity.

- **Your lifestyle doesn't allow it:** I travel often and find it difficult to maintain my fasting schedule on flight days. TRE or a 5:2 regimen can be frustrating for people who spend hours on the road, do shift work, or have more than one job. Intermittent fasting is still an option but will require adaptations from time to time to be effective and sustainable.

THE SCIENCE OF INTERMITTENT FASTING

Fasting is more than just going without food for set periods; it affects specific processes in your body. The power of fasting can be harnessed to reduce risk factors for various diseases and convey a myriad of other benefits, too. Let's dive deeper into how TRE impacts metabolism, hormones, cellular health, and longevity.

The Effects of Fasting on Metabolism and Hormones

Enzymes and hormones drive the metabolic pathways in your body. "Metabolism" simply refers to all the processes involved in converting the food you eat into energy. These include burning calories and storing what's left over as energy reserves.

Your body gets energy from two dietary sources: glucose and fatty acids.

The glucose circulating in your blood after consumption is a ready-to-use energy source. Extra glucose is stored as glycogen and released into the bloodstream if you get hungry or need energy. Once the glycogen stores are gone, your body will burn fat, which is ideal.

In times of desperation, skeletal muscles in your arms, legs, and trunk can become an alternate fuel source. However, we want to spare the muscles and burn the fat. This concept will be our intermittent fasting goal and mantra: "Spare the muscles, burn the fat!"

The fat from your meal is converted and stored in your body as fatty acids and cholesterol. Those acids will remain stored until needed, such as when your blood glucose levels run low; fasting creates such a scenario.

When there isn't enough glucose in the bloodstream to provide energy for physiologic processes, the liver will initiate a series of actions to convert fatty acids into ketones. Those ketones will fuel your body and brain.

Repeated episodes of fasting and fat burning will cause weight to decrease. Fat deposits around the organs, trunk, arms, and hips will shrink, and the body will have a trimmer appearance.

Prolonged fasting also enhances the release of serotonin. This hormone transmits messages between nerve cells in different parts of your body, including the brain. Those messages help with mood, digestion, wound healing, sexual desire, and bone health (Cleveland Clinic, 2022).

The Effects of Fasting on Cellular Health and Longevity

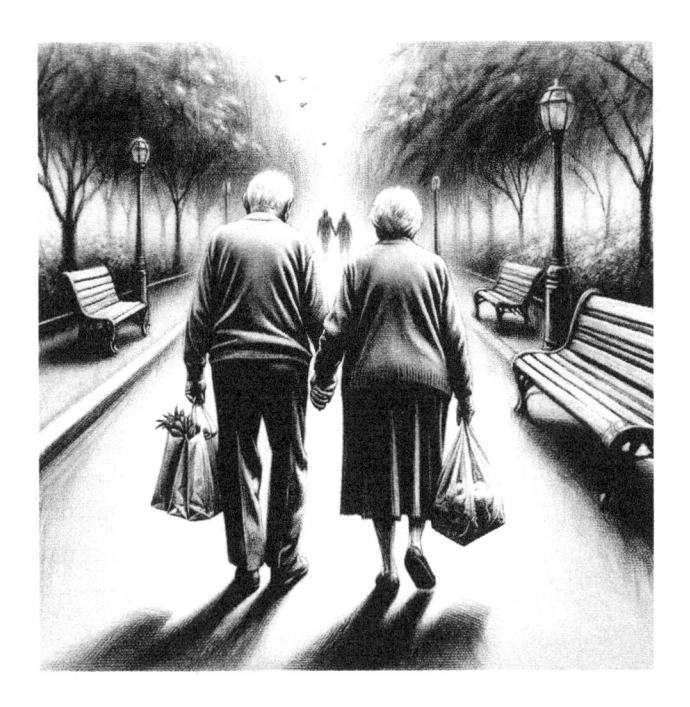

Though aging is a natural process, lifestyle and diet greatly determine the rate at which age-related changes manifest. Healthy diets can slow down the unfavorable biological aspects that signal advancing years, increasing longevity.

Here's something else to consider: The biological processes in your body release molecules called free radicals that can damage healthy cells. Ideally, your body's natural defenses would remove the free radicals as they form.

However, if the body lacks protective antioxidants, free radicals will accumulate. The build-up of these damaging particles causes oxidative stress, which speeds aging. Intermittent fasting helps to reduce the imbalance between antioxidants and free radicals.

Another way fasting enhances longevity is by protecting you from age-related ailments. Naturally, your immune system weakens as you get older. Some essential metabolic processes for survival also slow down, including the rate of cell regeneration and food digestion.

The heart muscle becomes less efficient, skin thins out, gums recede, tastebuds fade, and other processes decline with aging. All these factors will make your body more vulnerable to conditions such as heart disease, cancer, diabetes, and Alzheimer's disease.

Intermittent fasting can function as a reset by allowing the body the time it needs away from caloric intake to rest and recover.

At the cellular level, some of the benefits of intermittent fasting are tied to the specific type of fast and the foods consumed. A healthy diet enhances the fasting experience and maximizes outcomes. Rest and exercise also play an important role in cellular health and shouldn't be overlooked.

Specific Benefits

Fasting offers many benefits, even if you only follow a plan for a few weeks or months. The following checklist will help keep your eyes on the prize. Intermittent fasting

- improves the biological processes in your body
- increases longevity
- helps you to lose and manage weight
- optimizes hormone function
- reduces susceptibility to chronic diseases associated with aging
- improves mental clarity
- contributes to increased fitness

- enhances gut health and digestion

This chapter gave you an overview of what intermittent fasting is all about and how it impacts various body functions. You also gained a working knowledge of the most common fasting regimens. We saw that intermittent fasting isn't for everyone - it can aggravate chronic conditions if not done carefully.

Contact your healthcare provider before starting a fasting regimen, especially if you have underlying conditions. In the next chapter, we'll discuss the steps involved in preparing to fast and clarify some common misperceptions about intermittent fasting.

PREPARING TO FAST

Women often embark on an intermittent fasting or diet plan independently or without enough facts to inform their decisions, assuming that doing so is harmless. What we don't know can hurt us! Hidden illnesses may impact or be impacted by fasting.

Consider the prevalence of the Western diet and its globalization coupled with increasingly sedentary lifestyles. As a result of this diet, many people have associated conditions, including heart disease and cancer, but don't know it.

Hypertension and diabetes are just two examples of global health conditions that can exist for years without any symptoms. Liver and kidney disease are also widespread, and both progressively worsen under the radar for years before anyone is aware.

As discussed in the previous chapter, fasting will change how your body uses energy. Such alterations may aggravate or worsen an existing health condition. This possibility underscores the need to understand what intermittent fasting can and cannot do and to investigate if it's safe for you before starting a fasting regimen.

I've got you covered! The following sections will equip you to create a safe and realistic fasting plan that you can sustain for life.

COMMON MISPERCEPTIONS ABOUT FASTING

We'll start this chapter by looking at some of the misperceptions that can derail and frustrate your intermittent fasting experience (Nazish, 2021).

You Could Faint: Some people think that fasting drives your body into starvation mode, which can make you faint; this isn't true. To begin starving, you've got to go without caloric intake for more than 24 hours.

Earlier, I mentioned some of the most common types of intermittent fasting. None of them requires you to refrain from eating for more than 24 hours.

You'll Develop New Health Conditions: This misunderstanding comes from the idea that intermittent fasting reduces the rate of metabolism, which is true. However, as you consume fewer calories, your blood glucose, carbohydrate stores, and weight will also lower. The benefits far outweigh any concerns about developing a new condition because of reduced metabolism.

Nevertheless, when you fast for the first time, you'll feel tired and different. Fatigue associated with intermittent fasting often disappears after about ten days or so. Also, your mental health and focus will improve as you continue the practice.

Intermittent Fasting Primarily Involves Skipping Breakfast: Fasting schedules are flexible, and skipping breakfast is unnecessary. As a matter of practicality, it's better to eat breakfast and end your eating window early in the evening than to miss that morning meal.

The Eating Window Is Time To Make Up For Missed Calories: This idea is false and misguided; resist the urge to overindulge. Doing so defeats the purpose of the fasting period and is self-sabotaging. Instead, try to consume healthy foods during your eating window.

You Should Cut Down On Water Intake When Fasting: Nothing could be further from the truth! Though it's easy to forget to hydrate when you're not eating, your body needs water during fasting. Be intentional about hydrating throughout the entire day.

PRE-FASTING EVALUATION

At this point, you should already see the value of a health check before starting a fasting regimen. If for no other reason, you'll want to know if you have an undiagnosed condition that fasting can aggravate. A thorough assessment will reveal your baseline level of health and allow you to set goals that are directly and indirectly tied to the scale.

A pre-fasting evaluation may find that your weight gain or weight loss struggle is due to a condition that needs to be addressed first. This is especially true if you've previously tried to manage your weight without effect.

Essential Lab Tests

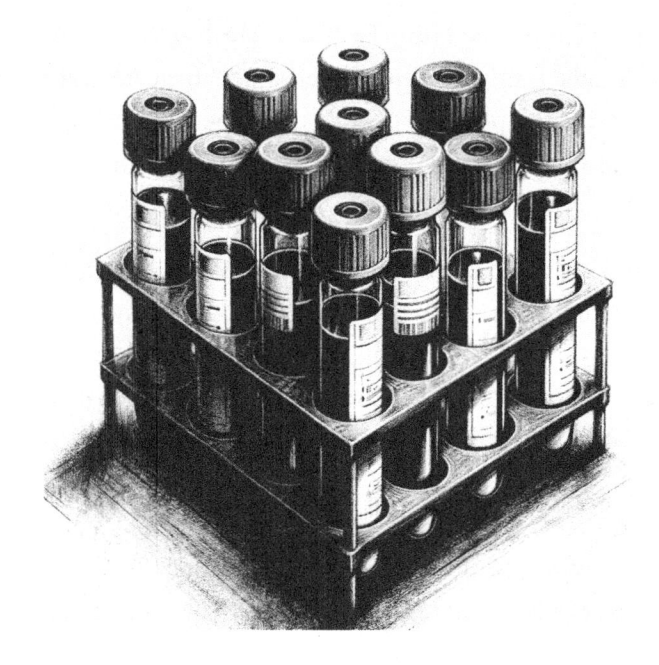

Regardless of why you want to start with intermittent fasting, some lab tests are worth considering at the outset. Lab results can help guide your decisions about what to eat and which fasting interval to choose. Blood tests include

- **Insulin profile, fasting sugar, and A1c:** These tests help you to know if you are diabetic or not. High levels of insulin in your body can cause an increase in body weight. This is because high insulin levels prevent fat from being broken down, allowing it to accumulate.

The fasting sugar level measures intake in the previous 24 hours. The hemoglobin A1c, known simply as "A1c", gives an average of your sugar levels over the previous three months.

- **Iron:** Iron deficiency interferes with your metabolism and lowers energy, leaving you exhausted. It's essential to correct iron deficits before you begin intermittent fasting.
- **Vitamin B12:** This water-soluble vitamin plays a role in carbohydrate, protein, and fat metabolism. Deficiency can cause you to feel weak, dizzy, and short of breath or cause slower metabolism and gut-related issues. Such symptoms can interfere with your intermittent fasting experience and outcomes.
- **Lipid profile:** This lab test looks at low-density lipoproteins (LDL), high-density lipoproteins (HDL), and triglycerides. LDLs are called "bad cholesterol"; HDLs are the good guys.

The liver uses triglycerides to make cholesterol. Even with low cholesterol intake, your LDL could be elevated if your diet is high in saturated fats such as butter and fatty red meat.

- **Vitamin D:** This vitamin plays an essential role in almost all physiologic processes and is vital to cell membrane composition. Deficiencies are widespread, even for people who live in sunny areas.
- **Thyroid levels:** A general thyroid panel checks thyroid stimulating hormone (TSH), thyroxine (T4), and triiodothyronine (T3). High TSH and low to normal T4 and T3 levels suggest that the thyroid gland is not doing its job well in regulating metabolism. This is a common cause of weight gain.
- **Sex hormone levels:** Some women who struggle with weight gain for years have undiagnosed or improperly managed polycystic ovary syndrome (PCOS). This condition is characterized by higher insulin and

testosterone levels, which can contribute to weight gain. PCOS increases the risk for metabolic disorders in and post-menopause.

As you can see, addressing health concerns and conditions starts with knowing your health status and lab levels. Barring any abnormal findings or contraindications, you'll be able to start with intermittent fasting.

TIPS FOR MENTALLY PREPARING FOR THE FASTING JOURNEY:

Evaluate arguments for or against intermittent fasting so you can reconcile them in your mind. What does the research show? What other information is available, and is it from a reputable source? Such an awareness boosts your mental preparedness and confidence in adopting the practice.

The last thing you want to do is start an intermittent fasting plan when you are still unsure if it can help you achieve your goals. Talk to your healthcare provider about the pros and cons and any reservations you have about fasting before getting started.

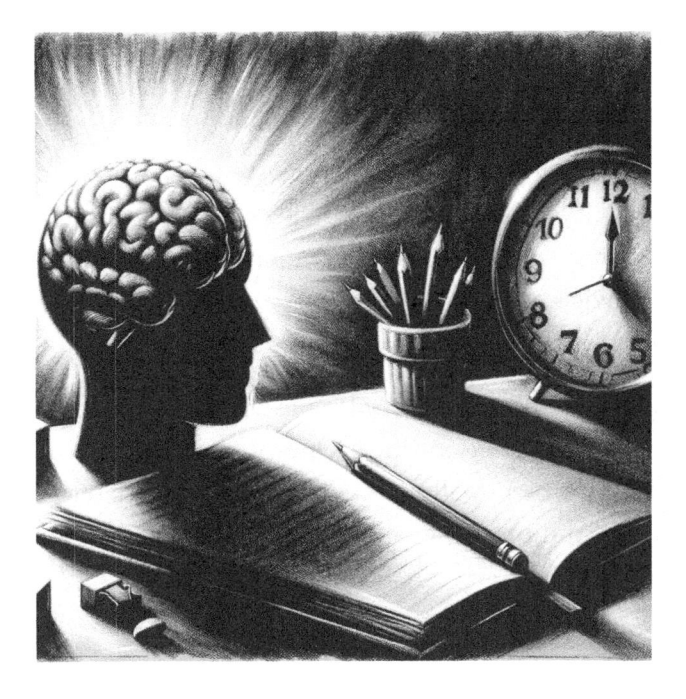

Seven Essential Questions

Consider the following questions before starting a fasting regimen:

1. What obstacles will you need to overcome to succeed at intermittent fasting?
2. How will you address hunger and cravings?
3. Will you prepare different meals in your home to accommodate others?
4. Are you comfortable cooking for others while you're not eating?
5. Who buys the groceries or has the final say on what goes in the basket?
6. What is your grocery budget - can you afford high-quality foods?

7. How will you navigate fasting during holidays, gatherings, and vacations?

It's best to plan for all of these things well in advance. Don't get discouraged if you don't have all the answers—this is where a support system pays off. Veteran intermittent-fasters will have plenty of advice to offer, so reach out and make the most of your connections.

I've compiled a table with everyday obstacles and solutions to help as you prepare for the journey. One of the strategies relates to caloric deficit, which we'll discuss in greater detail later on. I hope you find the solutions invaluable in formulating your fasting plan.

Table 1. Common obstacles and how to address them

Obstacle	Solution
You're the only person fasting at home	• Prepare your meals beforehand and eat with the family • Eat the same foods as the family but in smaller portions
You can't determine portion sizes	• Use a macro app for portion sizes and to track food intake • Read food labels • keep portion-sized scoops inside the food container and use them when preparing and plating your food
You're not sure what to buy at the grocery store	• Make a grocery list before going, and stick to it, always • Include a large variety of fruits, root and tuber vegetables, nuts, whole grains, legumes, fats, lean proteins, fish • Steer clear of prepackaged and processed foods
You had an "off" day	• Increase your caloric deficit over the next four days (if you went over by 500 calories, then your new daily caloric deficit will be 125 for each of four days) • Do a water, broth, vegetable, protein, and fruit day (avoid high-carb fruits and vegetables, bread, pasta, rice, potatoes, and other simple-carbohydrate foods)
You're traveling or working on the road and food choices are limited	• Pre-plan and pack healthy foods and snacks • Order the children's meal instead of the adult meal size • Select the lowest calorie, least processed meal options • Remove one or both slices of the bread/bun, half the fries/potatoes/rice or other carbohydrate in the meal • Drink water only; no juice, soda, or alcohol • Select salads without croutons; only use half the dressing • Select lean protein, high fiber meals • Select foods in their natural state (e.g. baked potato, not fries) • Have your last meal no less than three hours before bed • Go for a walk, exercise or increase your physical activity level to burn off some of the calories you consumed
You're going out for a meal	• Check the menu beforehand; select heart-friendly options • Order healthy appetizers instead of entrees • Share an entree • Divide the meal and take half of it to go • Select the lowest fat, carbohydrate, and calorie menu options • Limit or avoid alcoholic drinks, soda, juice, dessert

BUILDING A STRONG FOUNDATION

There are three macronutrients (macros) that all humans need: Carbohydrates, proteins, and fats. The term "macro" means that these nutrients are required in more significant amounts than others.

Carbohydrates are the primary energy source but are not all the same. In fact, we can even classify carbohydrates as either good or bad.

Carbohydrates from unprocessed foods like vegetables, grains, and fruits are good. Those that come from processed foods, including baked goods and products with added sugars, are bad.

The natural aging process is characterized by a weakening immune system, slow metabolism, and reduced lean muscle mass. The rate at which these changes occur is higher when dietary protein intake is inadequate.

Fish, eggs, dairy products, tofu, poultry, lentils, and beans are some of the protein-rich foods to include in your diet to ensure that you are getting enough of this macro. Nuts, asparagus, and other vegetables are excellent protein sources with low-calorie profiles.

There's a misperception that all fats are bad, but that's false. Dietary fats are needed to manufacture hormones and contribute to hormonal balance. Moreover, saturated fats are associated with better cognitive abilities.

Whole foods such as avocados, fatty fish, olives, seeds, and nuts will give your post-menopausal body the healthy fat it needs for better health. Extra virgin olive oil is an excellent fat, as are avocado and coconut oils. Consume dietary fats in moderation.

Calculating Your Macros

A balanced diet should contain all the macronutrients; too little or too much of any will be problematic. This is why it helps to know your ideal macro ratios and how they are calculated without getting lost in the weeds.

Macro calculations take into account your metabolism, activity level, and individual health goals; let's look at this in more detail. Feel free to skip this section if numbers bore or frustrate you. As they say, "There's an app for that!"

Step 1: Determine Your Basal Metabolic Rate (BMR)

The BMR is the number of calories your body requires to perform basic activities such as breathing, regulating temperature, and sleeping.

Several online BMR calculators are available, such as www.calculator.net/bmr-calculator.html.

These online tools determine your BMR based on age, weight, height, and gender and can quickly estimate your daily calorie needs. Feel free to find one, use it, and make a note of your BMR.

Step 2: Determine Your Total Daily Energy Expenditure (TDEE)

Energy use or expenditure largely depends on your daily activity level. According to Kallmyer (2019), if you are

- sedentary (little to no exercise): TDEE is your BMR x 1.2
- mildly active (light exercise or sports 1–3 days per week): TDEE = BMR x 1.375
- moderately active (exercise or sports 3–5 days a week): TDEE = BMR x 1.55
- very active (intense exercise or sports 6–7 days a week): TDEE = BMR x 1.725
- extremely active (high-intensity exercises or sports): TDEE = BMR x 1.9

Your TDEE will be equal to the number of calories that you should consume daily. However, you'll need to create a daily calorie deficit to lose weight.

A deficit of 500 calories is perfect for safe weight loss.

If your TDEE was 2,000 calories, your daily calorie consumption to lose weight would be 1,500. Using this example, the TDEE minus 500 calories is your ideal daily calorie intake (IDCI).

Step 3: Determine Macro Percentages

If you type "macro calculator" into the search bar of your browser, different online options will appear. Some of these calculators are free, while others have additional requirements or costs before you can access them.

Regardless of which one you choose, the calculators tend to agree on the ranges of macronutrient requirements for women like you and me who are over 50.

With that in mind, your daily calories should be divided to include

- 45%–65% carbohydrates.
- 20% –35% proteins.
- 20%–35% fats.

Start with 45% carbohydrates, 30% proteins, and 25% fats. I'm recommending the lowest intake of carbs because this macronutrient usually gets us women into trouble. Think back on the typical dinner plate: we tend to cover about half or more with rice, pasta, noodles, potatoes, or bread, right?

Note that one gram of carbohydrates provides four calories, one gram of protein provides four calories, and one gram of fat provides nine calories. We'll use these numbers shortly.

Step 4: Calculate Macro Grams

Macro grams are determined by multiplying the IDCI by the percentage of each macro. Using an IDCI of 1,500 per day and a goal macronutrient ratio of 45% carbohydrates, 30% proteins, and 25% fats, your calculations will be as follows:

- 1,500 cal x 0.45 = 675 cal

  675 cal ÷ 4 calories per gram = 168.75 g of carbs.

- 1,500 cal x 0.30 = 450 cal

  450 cal ÷ 4 calories per gram = 112 g of protein.

- 1,500 cal x 0.25 = 375 cal from fats

375 cal ÷ 9 calories per gram = 42 g of fats.

Write down the gram values you found for each macronutrient or enter them into your fasting or macro app.

- Carbohydrates_____
- Proteins_____
- Fats_____

Keep in mind that these calculations are just general guidelines. You'll need to modify your macros to find the best ratio based on your health factors, preferences, goals, home or work schedule, and social and family needs. Try to stay within the recommended minimum to maximum percentages.

If you still feel a bit confused, don't worry. Macros are such an important concept that we will see it again in Chapter 4, with sample tables to help you keep track of things.

Be careful not to go too low on your carbs; speaking from experience, it's a bad idea!

When I started fasting to lose weight, I tried to drop my carbohydrates down to 20%, and I was miserable! The task of sticking to that goal led to an obsession that was stressing me out! Eventually, I decided that the anxiety was counterproductive, and I raised my carbohydrate intake to about 35%.

My ideal carbohydrate macro percent is 35 and not 45 as a result of a lot of trial and error. I've been fasting intermittently long enough to know that bread and baked goods are my kryptonite. My mind is sharper, and I feel most energetic when my carbohydrate intake is no more than 35%.

Give yourself time to learn what works best and safest for you. Generally speaking, you'll be fine at whatever macro percentages you choose if you notice that you are achieving your health goals while staying healthy, energetic, and motivated.

FIND THE BEST METHOD FOR YOU

Most online sources say that women over 50 should adopt the 18:6 schedule, so that's what I did. However, I was working in a clinic while trying out the six-hour eating window and was constantly on the move.

With a start time of 8:30 a.m., I was getting lightheaded by 10 a.m. I eventually switched to a 16:8 schedule, which worked much better.

When I got a new job and found myself sitting for most of my workday, I realized that my digestion and metabolism had slowed. It was taking me longer to process proteins than when I started my fasting journey five years earlier.

After some experimentation, I shifted to a 14:10 schedule most days. Intermittently, I will fast for as long as 18 to 20 hours; this mix is a perfect fit for me at present.

Each of us has a different routine. Finding what works best for you and changing as life events dictate is the best way to approach intermittent fasting. This is especially true if you plan to make fasting a life-long practice.

This chapter reviews the different fasts for you to consider based on your unique needs, focusing on the TRE and 5:2 regimens. We'll explore their benefits, customization options, and tips for incorporating them into daily routines.

TIME-RESTRICTED EATING

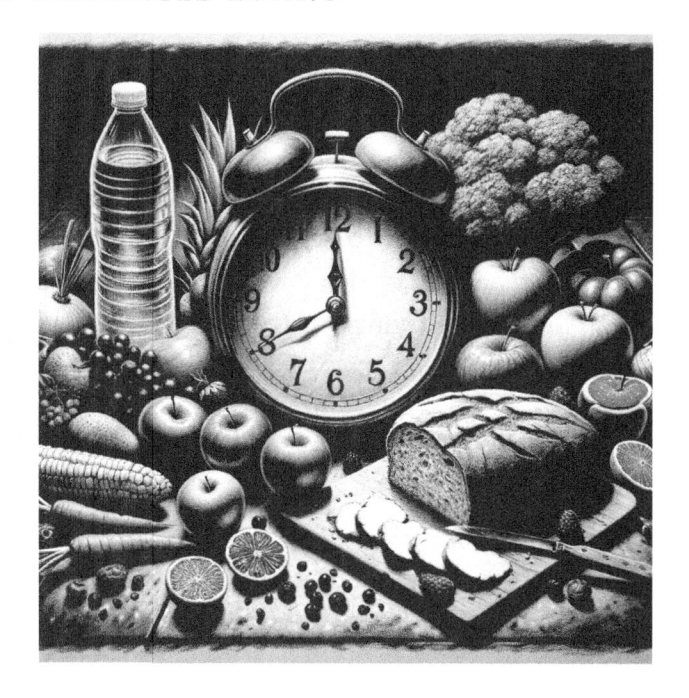

As previously mentioned, TRE is a fasting plan that restricts caloric intake to a specific time during the day. It has many variations, including 12:12, 14:10, 16:8, and 18:6.

One of the most common examples of the TRE regimen is the 16:8. Let's look at some of the benefits of this method and why it might be a great starting point for you. The 16:8 fast

- **Promotes fat burning:** You can burn fat for up to four hours by triggering ketosis around your 12th hour of fasting. This interval aids weight loss and protects you from chronic diseases exacerbated by the accumulation of fatty tissue.
- **Improves digestion and nutrient absorption**: A 16-hour fasting interval can benefit your gut health and overall well-being because it provides enough time to break down and properly absorb nutrients. With complete digestion, there will be less likelihood of bloating and discomfort.

When your gut is happy, your brain, organs, and joints are happy.

- **Matches any lifestyle:** The 16:8 fits your schedule and needs, allowing you to eat during your work day if your shift is only eight hours long. It also eliminates the mental gymnastics of meal planning because you can time your meals with traditional break times at work.

Consider an 8 a.m. to 4 p.m. or 9 a.m. to 5 p.m. work day: You could break your fast at 9 or 10 a.m, have lunch at noon or 1 p.m., and dinner between 5 p.m and 6 p.m. A substantial breakfast, moderate lunch, and light dinner will align with just about any weight loss goal.

If your work environment is not conducive to this strategy, move to a 12:12 or 14:10 regimen or find a middle-ground solution with a 13:11 or 15:9 schedule.

If your shift is 10 to 12 hours long, a tiny part of your fasting time will definitely fall within your day. Imagine you work from 7 a.m. to 7 p.m.; you could let two fasting hours fall at the beginning and end of your shift.

For an overnight 8-hour shift, try scheduling your fasting and eating times as though you're not a shift worker. Eat within one to two hours of arrival at work; take lunch about four hours later, then try to eat dinner at least three hours before bed.

A similar strategy could apply when traveling or doing something that keeps you away from home. Plan to start your day with two hours of fasting and end your eating window as early in the evening as is practical.

Making Time-Restricted Eating Work: Tips and Protein Sparing

When incorporating TRE into your daily routine, choose a sustainable plan by adopting a strategy that fits your grocery list and lifestyle well. To ensure success, shift your focus from short to long-term gains. I have a few additional tips to help with this process:

- **Stay hydrated:** Drink water throughout the day, aiming for at least eight cups (64 oz) or up to half of your body weight in ounces. Include herbal teas or unsweetened beverages in your fluid intake measurement. Adequate hydration aids digestion, metabolism, and overall well-being, making it an important aspect of successful TRE.
- **Eat a balanced diet:** Select a variety of foods from all food groups in proper portions, including eggs, tofu, fish and lean protein, fruits, vegetables, whole grains, and healthy fats. A balanced diet provides essential nutrients for overall health while supporting digestion and weight management.
- **Ensure adequate amounts of protein in your meals:** This macronutrient helps build and repair tissues and gives a

feeling of fullness. You're more likely to stick to your fasting plan if you don't feel weak and hungry all the time.

Women often encounter difficulties in obtaining sufficient protein, and I know this from personal experience. Further, with digestion slowing as we age, it can be tough to break down animal proteins; the process may take over four hours.

In my case, I can't go to bed within three hours of eating animal protein unless I recline at a 45-degree angle for the first one to two hours of sleep. Otherwise, I experience a lot of indigestion throughout the night.

Intermittent fasting can potentially lead to a loss of lean muscle mass during intervals of hunger beyond 24 hours. Just because the scale says weight is going down doesn't mean it's healthy weight loss.

When you start a fasting regimen, safeguard your muscle bulk by ensuring adequate protein intake. Recall our mantra: Spare the muscles, burn the fat!

A notable study by Yasuda et al. (2020) highlighted the importance of evenly distributing protein intake throughout the day, based on a concept known as protein sparing. This strategy is more advantageous for muscle maintenance and synthesis than consuming a large amount of the macro in just one or two meals.

Protein sparing also ensures a steady supply of amino acids—the building blocks of proteins—for the body to utilize throughout the day. Space out protein intake over three or more meals or snacks every three to four hours for best results.

THE 5:2 DIET AND VARIATIONS

For those who want to try the 5:2 diet, plan to significantly restrict calories on designated fasting days. The recommended maximum daily caloric intake is 500, leading to a substantial weekly calorie deficit depending on your weight, nutritional intake, and activity level.

You can experience fast and noticeable weight loss if you follow a healthy diet on the non-fasting days. Incorporate exercise to speed up the process.

Make fluid intake a priority on both fasting and non-fasting days. Pay attention to your body and drink more water if your urine is dark yellow or smells.

The same concerns apply if you're constipated, thirsty, or your skin is losing elasticity. Pinch the skin of your forearm for about two to three seconds, then let it go. If it stays tented, you're probably dehydrated. Ideally, it should quickly return to its resting position.

Be cautious about your food choices on your non-fasting days to ensure you stay within your macronutrient targets. Prioritize whole foods as they provide essential vitamins, minerals, and other building blocks for optimal health.

Customizing the 5:2 Diet

It's effortless to adapt the 5:2 diet to suit your lifestyle, vacation plans, outings with family and friends, and exercise routines. Here are some tips to help:

- **Create a shopping list:** Focus on low glycemic index (low sugar content) foods, such as whole grains, non-starchy vegetables, fruits, lean meats, poultry, fish, eggs, beans, and tofu. Remember to include anti-inflammatory options like berries and leafy greens; add healthy fats such as avocados and extra virgin olive oil.

Steer clear of white bread, pasta, rice, and potatoes, processed and pre-packaged foods, sugar, and most sugar substitutes.

- **Meal prep:** This time-saving practice ensures nutritious meals and snacks are readily available for fasting and non-fasting days. You can streamline your process by batch-cooking proteins, grains, and vegetables in advance.

Dividing your food into convenient meal prep containers allows for effortless grab-and-go options. It helps you adhere to your 5:2 fasting plan more effectively.

- **Plan for social events:** Consider adjusting your non-eating days around your obligations. If you have an upcoming special occasion or gathering centered around food, schedule it as a regular eating day.
- **Account for exercise:** Save intense workouts for days when you have regular calorie intake. Attempting them on fasting days may lower energy levels and increase your risk for dangerously low blood sugar (hypoglycemia).
- **Determine frequency and sustainability:** Decide how often you want to incorporate fasting days into your routine, such as once or twice a month. If you want to fast more frequently but find the 5:2 method too challenging, consider transitioning to a TRE regimen.
- **Be creative with your food choices:** Consider nutrient-dense soups, casseroles, and shakes with a low-calorie

count. I love to soft cook a variety of vegetables, purée them, then return them to their pot water to make a very low-calorie, delicious soup.

Soups and shakes offer a great way to increase your intake of vegetables, even if you don't particularly enjoy biting into or chewing them. You'll find a recipe for my favorite vegetable soup in Chapter 4.

Managing Hunger and Energy Levels on Fasting Days

When following the 5:2 diet, it may seem impossible to address hunger and maintain energy levels during those 500-calorie days. Implementing effective strategies and making mindful choices can help you stay on track. Here are some helpful tips:

- **Add some flavor:** Sip on herbal teas, black coffee, flavored sparkling water, apple cider vinegar water, lemon water, and similar beverages during your fasting windows to provide a sense of satisfaction without adding extra calories.
- **Eat filling foods:** Prioritize foods that are rich in both fiber and lean or plant-based protein. Cruciferous vegetables and whole grains are just a couple examples of wholesome products that take longer to digest and leave you feeling satiated longer during your fasting hours.
- **Spread out your meals:** On fasting days for the 5:2 regimen, there are only two meals: ideally, one should contain about 200 calories, and the other should have about 300 calories.

Though I haven't found consensus in the research, consuming the calories over a maximum six to eight-hour window makes sense.

This approach would maximize fat burning while helping to manage hunger more effectively throughout the day.

Consuming three to five smaller meals or snacks is possible if you stay within the 500-calorie restriction. For me, it might look like this: 100-calorie vegetable soup for breakfast, lunch, and dinner; two 100-calorie protein snacks in between, and drinking only water with apple cider vinegar.

- **Distract yourself:** Learn to divert your attention from food to manage hunger on your 500-calorie days by engaging in activities that occupy your mind. Stay busy with hobbies, work, or other tasks that take your mind off your stomach.

In this chapter, we explored the most common intermittent fasting approaches. I've offered many tips to increase your chances of success.

Now, let's move on to the next chapter, discussing the importance of balanced nutrition in conjunction with intermittent fasting. We'll also explore creating a well-rounded eating plan that supports overall health and weight loss goals.

UNLOCK THE POWER OF BALANCED NUTRITION

About 16 years ago, I was 15 pounds overweight, and my flabby parts had a lot of jiggle. I crafted a workout routine to burn 1,000 calories on each trip to the gym, five days weekly. I also dropped my daily caloric intake down to 1,200 calories.

My diet consisted of a ton of vegetables, some fruits, high-quality protein, and limited simple carbohydrates. Back then, I knew nothing about macros but was sticking to my diet and exercise plans like a pro!

Six months later, I hadn't dropped a single pound. If my waist and arms got trimmer or more toned, I couldn't tell. I was so disappointed and discouraged that I stopped everything.

It was baffling as to why my body refused to let the fat, flab, and weight go. I later realized that my diet didn't have enough protein or carbs to support my intense exercise. I was fighting a losing battle.

It's one thing to trim calories, but if your nutrition isn't balanced, the weight won't come off. Or, changes on the scale will be due to reduced lean muscle mass and lost water weight. As many of you have discovered, with fast and fad diets, weight loss medications, and surgeries, you'll just gain the pounds back if the method used to shed them isn't sustainable.

Nevertheless, my story ends well: After adopting a balanced diet with adequate protein and water, my weight started reflecting my efforts. I am confident you can achieve the same success with additional guidance.

NUTRITION BASICS

The easiest way to upgrade your nutritional intake is to eat whole foods and avoid processed foods. Include a wide variety of vegetables (naturally high in fiber) to get the most nutrients, as some may excel in one area but lack in another.

Consider taking a high-quality multivitamin if you're worried about getting your vitamins and minerals. Look for a pharmaceutical-grade multivitamin for women with a stamp on the packaging or bottle indicating that it has passed rigorous, standardized lab testing. A good multivitamin should have little to no calories or fillers.

To increase your chances of getting the most nutrients at every meal, include two to three different types and colors of vegetables in an amount that covers half of your plate. Multiply the impact of your diet by adding one half to one full cup of various low-sugar fruits two to three times daily.

Exponentially multiply the nutritional impact of your meals by consuming three to four ounces of lean protein, tofu, other vegetable protein, or fatty fish (tuna, salmon, and others). Each meal will pack a powerful health punch if you include no more than about half a cup of whole grain or other complex carbohydrates.

Following these simple recommendations means you don't have to obsess about which food has what particular nutrient or worry about an unbalanced diet. However, many people find it challenging to cut down on simple carbohydrates. Here are a few strategies that can help:

- Measure your rice, pasta, noodle, yam, bread, and potato intake before putting it on your plate. Limit these carbs to no more than half a cup per meal. After one or two weeks, you'll know what that half-cup serving looks like without continuing to measure it.
- When eating a sandwich, make it open-faced to cut the bread down to half of your usual intake or wrap the sandwich contents in a large lettuce leaf and nix the bread
- Make a deal with yourself to finish all of your vegetables, protein, and a glass of water first before eating your carbohydrate.

Purge and Reload

When putting together your grocery list, start with a purge. I want you to be successful, and you want to be successful, right? It's impossible to achieve that goal if temptation hides behind your refrigerator, cabinet, and pantry doors. Here are a few tips to help achieve your goals:

- Throw out all opened processed food items that contain added salt or sugar
- Donate unopened items from your fridge and pantry that are processed or have added salt and sugar, including

canned goods. The idea is to avoid wasting food when people may benefit from what you donate because they don't have other options.

- Commit to buying a colorful variety of farm fresh or frozen fruits and vegetables; grass-fed and finished meats; quality tofu or other vegetable protein; wild-caught fish like salmon and tuna; whole grains like barley, wheat, and oats; complex carbohydrates like lentils, beans, quinoa, sweet potatoes, and yams; seeds like flax and chia; plain yogurt, kefir, kombucha; apple cider vinegar; extra virgin olive oil, avocado oil, coconut oil; snacks with no added sugar, salt or chemicals; spices like turmeric, cardamom, saffron, rosemary, sage, thyme, black pepper, cayenne pepper, and many others.
- Look to cultural cookbooks and recipes for healthy items to add to your list. You can also search online for more foods and spices to include in your stash.
- Prepare a week's worth of food in batches to help save money when shopping and prevent waste. Leftovers can be vacuum-packed and frozen.
- Try not to load up on cookbooks unless you like to do that sort of thing. It's so easy to search online for healthy recipes using the ingredients that you have on hand. Include an ethnicity in your query if you want recipes specific to a particular culture.

Make mealtimes easy and fun. Don't be afraid to try a new recipe or food on your own by using the tools you already have, such as your smartphone or computer.

DESIGNING NUTRIENT-DENSE MEALS

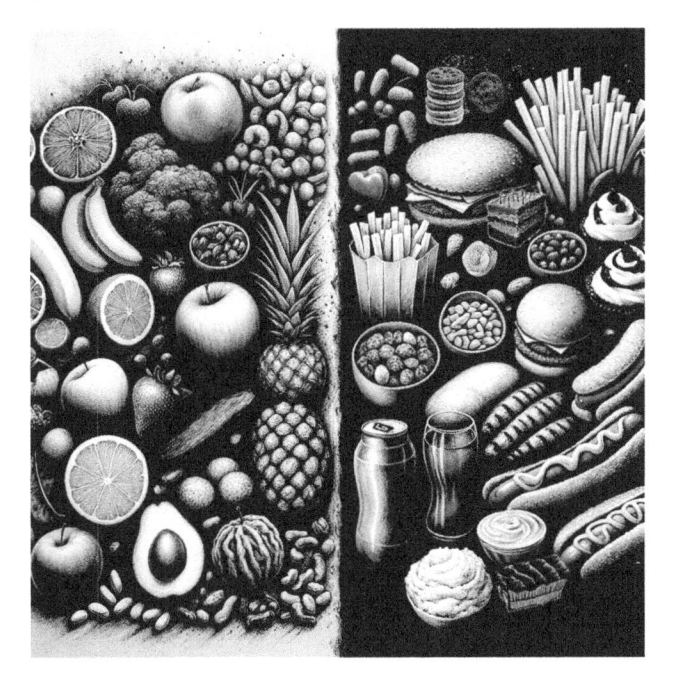

Eat foods that remember where they came from! For instance, apples *know* that they fell from a tree, but Apple Jacks have no clue how they came to be. Whole foods are your best bet.

Essential micronutrients such as iron, calcium, zinc, and folate are abundant in whole foods. The procedures involved in processing what we consume tend to reduce the available concentrations of these vital nutrients.

However, eating whole foods is only as good as monitoring your portion sizes. Too much of anything, even if it's healthy, is not good! For example, grapes are a delicious and natural snack, but one cup has the equivalent of over three teaspoons of sugar. A medium banana has almost four.

Stick to Your Macros

The macronutrients (macros) that comprise most of our daily intake are carbohydrates, fats, and protein. A helpful strategy is to keep simple carbohydrates to a minimum and eliminate unhealthy fats. Doing so will help lower your diet's glycemic index (GI) and inflammatory impact.

The higher the GI of a food, the more sugar it pumps into your system after consumption. Sugar can damage the delicate tissues of nerves and arteries, creating inflammatory changes that lead to disease.

Your body works harder to process complex carbohydrates like quinoa, beans, whole grains, and sweet potatoes than it does for simple carbohydrates. That extra effort of digestion burns calories.

Sample Tables to Help You Succeed

As you begin to refine your eating plan, you may need to take a few notes; the following tables should help. Customize each to suit your goals and lifestyle and update them monthly.

Table 2. Tracking Weight and Macros

Date of calculation			
Current weight			
Protein % and grams			
Fat % and grams			
Carb % and grams			
Daily calorie goal (aka IDCI)			

Table 3. Custom Grocery List - add as many lines as needed for shopping

Lean Proteins	Low Glycemic Index Fruits	Low Glycemic Index Vegetables	Low Glycemic Index Carbohydrates (potatoes, yams, noodles, breads, etc.)	Oil/Fat Options	Sugar and Snack Options

Table 4. Favorite Restaurants - Keep on hand for macro-friendly menu items

Restaurant Name	Appetizer(s)	Entree(s)	Dessert(s)	Drink(s)

Recipes and Meal Ideas

This section of the book offers meal ideas that you can use as a foundation. I prefer to prepare a batch of mains that I can modify for each meal, such as soups, grains, and vegetable blends. Experiment to see if my approach can fit your lifestyle, or explore other alternatives from friends, family, and intermittent fasting buddies.

The recipes below fit the food planning principles we've been discussing in previous chapters. Some include macro and calorie counts, but not all.

Nutritional Porridge Bowl

This porridge is a good breakfast option, enriched with berries, seeds, oats, and bananas. It's a nutrient-packed recipe that can boost the body and mind. Expect about 633 cal from these ingredients, in addition to 66 g of carbohydrates, 17 g of protein, and 19 g of fat (Good Food Team, n.d.). Split the yield into as many servings as needed to fit your macros.

Ingredients

- 1 ½ cups porridge oats
- ¾ cup frozen raspberries
- 1 tbsp chia seeds
- 2 tbsp almond butter
- 1 tbsp goji berries
- ½ banana cut into slices
- 3 ⅓ fl oz milk
- 15 fl oz water
- ½ orange, sliced
- juice of half an orange

Instructions

1. Place all the orange juice and half of the raspberries into a pan. Allow the pan contents to simmer for five minutes while the raspberries soften.

2. Add the water, milk, and oats to another pan. Cook on low heat while gently stirring.

3. Top with the fruit mixture you prepared in Step 1. Also, add the orange slices, remaining raspberries, goji berries, banana, chia seeds, and almond butter.

Mackerel Salad

Prepare this meal for lunch or dinner. The recipe contains spinach, rich in iron, manganese, magnesium, and folate. The mackerel in this recipe is a fantastic source of nutrients such as selenium, calcium, protein, phosphorus, zinc, and vitamins B6 and B12.

The vitamin B5 and copper from the mushrooms are an additional treat for your body. The same applies to the potassium and vitamin C found in tomatoes.

This recipe will give you a serving for one person. It comes with 280 cal, 15 g of carbohydrates, 28 g of protein, and 11 g of fat (Optimizing Nutrition, n.d.).

Ingredients

- 1 ¾ cups raw spinach
- 1 large tomato, ripe, uncooked, and sliced
- 3.4 oz canned and drained mackerel (feel free to substitute an alternative fish)
- 10 black olives
- ½ lemon
- ⅓ raw red pepper, cut to slices
- ½ small cucumber, cut to slices
- 1 tbsp jalapenos
- 8 snow peas, raw and sliced
- salt and pepper (to taste)

Instructions

1. Wash the vegetables and slice them into smaller salad pieces.
2. Place the seafood or fish on top of the vegetables
3. Squeeze the lemon juice on the fish and vegetables.
4. Sprinkle the pepper and salt to taste.

Nutrient-packed Vegetable Soup

This soup is my all-time favorite and personal recipe. I use it to get back on track after traveling or eating out. The recipe is excellent for people who don't like biting into vegetables.

Adapt this soup for breakfast by topping it with bacon, scrambled eggs, pepitas, roasted tomatoes, and bell peppers. It's also an excellent option for lunch or dinner; just add chopped, seasoned avocado, and grilled chicken or salmon. Shredded cheese, ground beef, sausage, tofu, and other meat substitutes offer alternatives.

This soup will take its coloring from the vegetable present in the greatest quantity. It has negligible fat and is naturally low in carbohydrates and calories.

The amount of soup produced will vary based on how thick or watery you prefer. My recipe below yielded 16 cups; its consistency was slightly more fluid than a smoothie. Use a high-quality, large-quantity blender for best results.

Ingredients

- 1 cup each of chopped kale, spinach, chayote, zucchini, broccoli, cauliflower, carrots, squash
- ½ cup each of chopped red peppers, yellow peppers, peas
- 2 garlic cloves

- ¼ cup onion
- 10-14 cups water (depending on the desired thinness or thickness of soup)
- salt (to taste)
- a pinch of turmeric and black pepper

Instructions

1. Put the chopped vegetables, garlic, and onion in a deep soup pot
2. Add cold water until it covers the vegetables by three to four inches.
3. Cover the pot, bring everything to a boil, then reduce the heat to medium.
4. Check the pot frequently; add water to cover the vegetables if needed.
5. Use a fork to pierce the carrots, broccoli stems, and chayote. Remove the pot from the heat once the fork passes through each easily.
6. Let the soup cool for about 20-30 minutes.
7. After the soup has cooled down, use a strainer spoon to remove all the soft-cooked vegetables and put them in the blender. Don't throw out the pot water! It contains all the water-soluble vitamins from the vegetables.
8. Add two to four cups of cold water to a large blender (64-ounce capacity) to cover the soft vegetables. If you don't have a large blender, just plan to purée the vegetables in small batches; add water to each batch as needed.
9. Use the pulse feature to purée the vegetables at high speed until the mixture has a smooth consistency. Periodically open the vent on the blender to let heat escape.
10. Return the purée to the original pot of water; stir the mixture and add salt, turmeric, and pepper to taste. Add

other seasonings as desired, and enjoy!

Veggie Hash

My brother makes a delicious vegetable hash that seems to be a pleaser for even the pickiest eaters. You can customize this dish for breakfast, lunch, or dinner. Below is the recipe for the basic hash; feel free to add or subtract vegetables for a wider variety of options.

It's great as a side dish, or it can also be the main entree: Simply toss it in with scrambled eggs, sausage, chopped chicken or steak, crumbled bacon, tofu, or fish. If desired, top the mixture with your favorite crushed nuts or shredded cheese. This recipe will serve three to four people.

Ingredients

- 1 cup each of fresh or frozen cauliflower, broccoli, zucchini, carrots
- ¼ cup onion and each of red, orange, green, and yellow bell peppers
- 1 garlic clove
- 2 tablespoons of extra virgin olive oil
- salt (to taste)
- A pinch of turmeric and black pepper

Instructions

1. Chop all vegetables, onions, and garlic, or use a food processor for fast results. The final size of each piece should be smaller than the diameter of a pea.
2. Preheat the olive oil in a large non-stick pan or wok.

3. Once the oil is hot, add the chopped vegetables and stir the mixture frequently.
4. Sautee for about five minutes for al dente or up to 10 minutes for a very soft consistency.
5. Add salt, turmeric, and black pepper to taste
6. Add a protein and enjoy!

Kale Pasta Sauce

This dish is not only nutrient-dense, it is also flavorful and quick to make. The fresh garlic lends the sauce its flavor, as does a small amount of fresh-squeezed lemon.

The kale pasta sauce has 146.9 cal and will serve five people. In addition to the micronutrients such as calcium, potassium, sodium, and vitamin C in this meal, you will also benefit from 2.6 g of carbohydrates, 1.6 g of protein, and 2.1 g of fat.

This dish takes about 33 minutes to make from start to finish, which is not bad for a freshly prepared delicious topper (Bell, 2022). The sauce pairs excellently with pasta, but there are other options: you can serve it over spaghetti squash or spiralized vegetables.

Alternatively, pour it over fish or chicken and add a side of risotto, quinoa, wild rice, salad, or vegetables. The choices are endless!

Ingredients

- 1 lemon, zested and juiced
- ¼ cup cold water
- 4 cups raw kale, chopped
- 1 garlic clove
- ⅓ cup extra virgin olive oil
- salt (to taste)

- pepper (a pinch)

Instructions

1. Preheat your oven to 350 ºF.
2. Add the cold water and chopped kale to an oven-safe baking dish.
3. Place the dish in the oven for 25 minutes.
4. Add the following ingredients to a blender: the cooked kale, lemon juice, garlic, extra virgin olive oil, salt, and lemon zest.
5. Process these ingredients until you see a smooth appearance.
6. Serve over your preferred protein, grain, or vegetable, and enjoy!

Fig Cookies

This fig dessert offers loads of fiber and nutrients essential to your health and mood. It's dairy and egg-free and packed with 120 cal, 14.4 g of carbohydrates, 3.8 g of protein, and 6.1 g of fat (Bell, 2023).

Ingredients

- 12 dried figs
- ½ cup smooth almond butter at room temperature
- 2 tsp pure vanilla extract
- 1 tsp baking powder
- 1 cup cassava flour (or mix ¾ cup cassava flour with ¼ cup regular flour) ¼ tsp salt
- 1 cup boiling water
- melted chocolate for drizzling on the cookies (optional)

Instructions

1. Roughly chop the figs after having removed the stems.
2. Add boiling water to a bowl before adding the chopped figs. Allow them to soak for about 30 minutes.
3. Preheat your oven to 375 °F.
4. Transfer all the bowl's contents to a blender. Also, add the vanilla extract, smooth almond butter, and salt. Process until you get a consistent mixture.
5. Mix the baking powder with the cassava flour in a separate bowl.
6. Then, add the blender contents to the bowl with the flour. Using your hands, mix and knead to incorporate the ingredients.
7. Create 12 balls from the dough. Line two sheet pans with parchment paper and place the dough balls on the sheet pans.
8. Flatten the dough into circular shapes using your fingers.
9. Bake for 17 minutes.
10. Drizzle melted chocolate on the cookies as an optional finishing touch. Refrigerate for 30 minutes before serving.

Green Smoothie

This nutrient-dense snack is loaded with healthy ingredients: antioxidants, vitamins B12, C, and K, and minerals such as potassium and copper. The recipe makes one serving in five minutes, with 99 cal, 23 g of carbohydrates, 2 g of proteins, and 1 g of fat (The Test Kitchen, 2013).

Ingredients

- 1 cup loosely packed, chopped, and stemmed kale
- 1 banana

- 1 cup ice cubes
- ½ peeled and chopped apple
- ½ cup almond milk

Instructions

Add all the ingredients to a blender and process until smooth. Enjoy!

HYDRATION AND INTERMITTENT FASTING

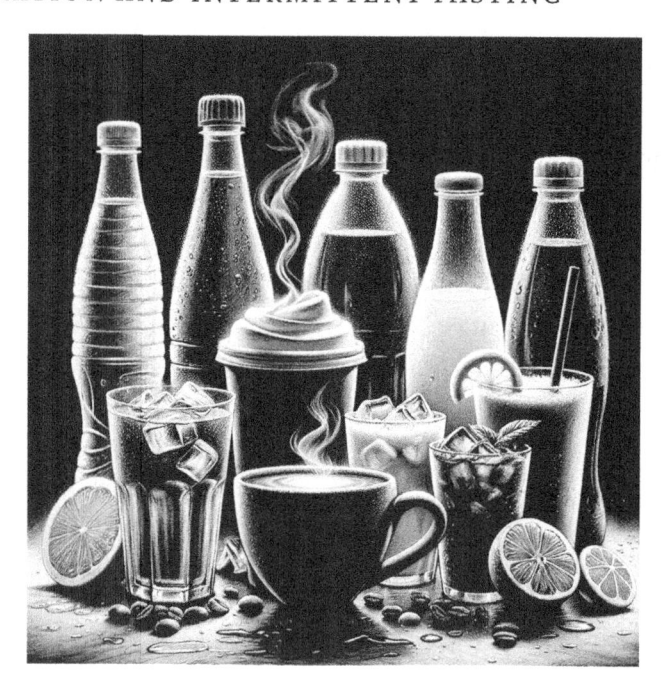

If drinking plain water is challenging, try flavoring it with apple cider vinegar (ACV), freshly squeezed lemon juice, or fruit and vegetable slices such as lemon, cucumber, and lime. There is a small caloric intake with lemon juice and zero calories with ACV; both accelerate fat burning.

I like to add just a few drops of citrus essential oil (labeled for internal consumption) to my water. Doing so gives me the flavor I'm looking for, but the caloric intake is negligible and doesn't kick me out of a fasting state.

Check if your fluid intake is adequate by looking at your urine and taking a whiff! Urine should have only a slight yellow color and little to no odor.

However, you may notice a metallic smell in your urine soon after adopting a nutrient-dense diet. This odor usually reflects increased protein intake—it's not necessarily a cause for concern.

See your healthcare provider for an evaluation as a precaution, especially if the color is dark and the odor is strong or foul.

There's no 'one size fits all' when it comes to fluid intake. Keep exploring to discover what suits you, and adopt a plan for hydration that will be comfortable and sustainable for the long haul.

Drinks to Include

There are other beverages to consider during your eating window, including fruit juices. While juicing is excellent, it can add a lot of calories, so keep portion sizes to about four ounces to avoid straying away from your macros.

Options include

- fresh squeezed or pressed orange, watermelon, pineapple, or carrot juice
- unsweetened teas
- coffee with coconut, almond, oat, cow, rice, or goat milk and the healthiest sweetener you can find if needed at all

Caramel macchiato lattes are delicious; I indulge about once a month, then make up for it by burning calories with a walk, moderately strenuous chores around the house or yard, or an otherwise very low-carb day. Find creative ways to stay on track after treating yourself and straying from your macros.

Drinks to Avoid

Empty calories will sabotage your weight loss efforts. A drink with 40 g of sugar, such as a can of soda or bottle of juice, has 10 or more teaspoons of sugar!

Try to stay away from

- Soda
- Drinks with added sugars - always check the label
- Drinks with artificial sweeteners, especially aspartame

Knowledge is power—this can't be emphasized enough. Understanding the concept of nutrition and hydration and how these two factors interrelate with intermittent fasting can help you achieve your desired results.

You may still hit a plateau even when you observe all the recommended fasting tips and tricks. We'll address this problem in great detail in the next chapter.

BREAK THROUGH BARRIERS, PLATEAUS, AND OBSTACLES

Our best-laid plans can get derailed—just like that!

My daughter loves to go out for lunch after church. I'm usually hungry by mid-Sunday, and I enjoy our time together, so I oblige whenever possible.

Recently, we went to a favorite restaurant, and I fully intended to order a salad. Once I started looking at the menu, the eggs, bacon, and home-fried potatoes were too tempting. I thought, no problem! I'll divvy up my meal, eat half now, and save the rest for later —NOT!

By the time I'd finished eating, I'd blown way past my macros for the day and had borrowed from Monday's allotment! While shuffling out of the restaurant, I came to the realization that my defenses are pretty low when my favorite comfort foods are within sight.

I stray from my fasting plan at least once a month, so I keep follow-up and contingency plans in place to get back on track within the next day or two. Is this something that you've been experiencing? If yes, this chapter has you covered. If you haven't gone through this yet, remember that to be forewarned is to be forearmed.

Slip-ups happen to everyone, regardless of age or how long you've been intermittent fasting. Don't be too hard on yourself when you have a momentary lapse. It's all about how quickly and successfully you can bounce back.

You have the strength and ability to overcome any obstacle that comes your way. Keep your eyes on the prize and stay motivated to achieve your health goals.

This chapter will cover strategies for managing hunger and cravings and tips for overcoming weight loss plateaus. Hopefully, you'll feel much more confident about your fasting plan after reading and applying what you learn in this part of the book.

DEALING WITH HUNGER AND CRAVINGS

First, review what happens when you eat: The chewed food moves from your mouth down through the esophagus and enters your stomach. The stomach acts like a balloon that stretches as it fills up. This expansion triggers nerves in your stomach to send messages to your brain.

The brain responds to those messages by causing a release of enzymes to break down the food. As the particles are digested, they move from your stomach to your small intestine, where nutrients are absorbed into your bloodstream.

After the initial digestion phase, the remaining bulk or bolus moves to your large intestine (colon). Water and electrolytes are absorbed and sent to your kidneys, where some of that fluid will become urine. The remaining solid waste in the colon becomes fecal matter and will eventually be eliminated from your body.

Hormones Associated With Hunger and Cravings

Let's look at some of the hormones involved with eating to better understand how the body processes food. This brief review will present opportunities for improvement in eating habits that can bolster success with intermittent fasting.

Ghrelin

Your brain works hard to balance the input it receives from different sources to keep your body functioning correctly. These sources of information include the hormones in your body, like ghrelin, whose role is to make sure you never go hungry.

Your empty stomach releases ghrelin, which stimulates your appetite until you eat something. This process ensures you have enough energy to fuel all your activities.

Ghrelin also causes your body to store energy in the form of fat as a backup in case you can't find food for a while. However, the more you eat, the more your body will store the extra fat.

It's essential to be aware of how much you eat and avoid over-consuming. Make healthy choices and practice portion control to prevent unwanted weight gain.

Also, distinguish between eating for health and eating as an emotional outlet; the latter will undoubtedly get you into trouble. Journaling your emotions when eating can help to reveal and reset your relationship with food; counseling can also help with this process.

With appropriate dietary corrections, ghrelin levels will reduce to normal, and fatty deposits will shrink.

Leptin

Fat cells in your adipose tissue release leptin, which helps balance how much you eat and the energy you burn. As you accumulate adipose tissue, leptin tells your brain you are not starving. Hence, you can stop eating. And, you can afford to burn off some of your fat stores.

Your weight stays within a healthy range when this system functions as designed. However, excess leptin is problematic.

Let me explain.

I once worked in a building where it seemed there was at least one false fire alarm every week! After a while, my coworkers and I became insensitive to the blazing sound; we simply ignored it as long as possible without risking a reprimand.

The fire truck would come, and we would reluctantly drag ourselves through the corridors and stairways until everyone was huddled at our designated waiting areas. We entertained one another and mumbled our discontent until it was time to march back to our respective workstations and tasks.

A similar response occurs in the presence of excess fatty tissue and leptin.

The ever-increasing levels of leptin become an annoyance that the brain ignores. In short, the brain becomes insensitive to leptin. This insensitivity partly explains why it's so difficult to stop eating when we're not truly hungry: Leptin is talking, but the brain isn't listening.

To restore the normal brain-leptin relationship, we've got to create a healthy eating plan and discipline ourselves to stick to it. By doing so, logic and reason will tell us when it's time to stop eating.

A balanced diet with careful attention to portion sizes is also essential. There's no need to obsess over portion sizes, but we do have to be mindful. Over time, the brain-leptin insensitivity will wane, and the struggle won't seem so unbearable.

Chocolate is my weakness. In the past, I used to eat two or three milk chocolate bars in a row without hesitation! I wore those delicacies on my abdomen, hips, and thighs for many years until I started intermittent fasting. Now, the intense sweet cravings are gone.

Whatever your kryptonite, if I can succeed, so can you!

Cholecystokinin

Cholecystokinin (CCK) is another vital hormone involved in digestion. Think of it as a traffic controller in your intestines: It coordinates the digestive process. When food enters the small intestine, CCK swings into action, telling the body to release digestive enzymes to break food down into molecules that it can absorb.

This hormone also slows food traffic from the stomach into the small intestine, giving the digestive enzymes enough time to do their job effectively. Once the food is adequately broken down, CCK pushes it from the small intestine to the large intestine.

A balanced diet helps your body respond naturally to the food you consume so that CCK can do its job well. Mindful eating, with regular pauses between mouthfuls, provides the time CCK needs to keep things moving at an ideal pace.

Acknowledging Hunger and Fullness Cues

Have you ever struggled to recognize when you've had enough to eat? It can be challenging to gauge your fullness accurately, leading to overeating, feeling uncomfortably stuffed, and hitting a plateau.

Susan Albers, a psychologist, explains that there's often a delay between physically satisfying your hunger and your brain registering the feeling of fullness (Cleveland Clinic, 2023). This delay can lead you to overconsume before your brain catches up with your stomach.

Various factors, including dopamine, peptide release, and muscle stretching in your stomach, signal fullness. Eating too quickly can interfere with this process.

Knowing when you're full is vital for your overall well-being. The human body has these fantastic cues we experience as hunger and fullness. Let's not ignore them or push them aside.

Here's a nifty trick to help gauge fullness: Reframe the idea of being "full" as being "satiated." When you're eating, ask yourself if you're still hungry or not. Eat only until you're satisfied, then stop.

Don't give in to urges to eat until you're bursting at the seams. Remember, it's all about finding that balance and listening to your body's signals. She who eats and walks away lives to eat another day, right?

There are several strategies to employ during both phases of intermittent fasting that can minimize overeating and hunger and prevent cravings. See if any of the following resonate with you:

Eat nutrient-dense foods: Choose low glycemic, anti-inflammatory foods that align with your macronutrient goals. These include berries, fatty fish, mushrooms, and vegetables with high fiber content to increase satiety.

Eat slower: Take your time while eating and practice mindful eating. After every three to five fork or spoonfuls, set your utensil down for a few minutes. Doing so allows your body to register feelings of satiety more accurately, preventing overeating.

Stay hydrated: Drink plenty of water, green tea, herbal teas, lemon water, and water with apple cider vinegar. Recall from Chapter 4 that lemon water and apple cider vinegar help your body burn fat.

Increase protein intake: Consuming adequate protein during your eating window helps promote satiety and reduce hunger. Protein sources such as meat, fish, eggs, or vegan alternatives provide a more sustainable feeling of fullness than protein shakes.

Go for healthy snacks and alternatives: Eat nuts, cheese, or meat strips when cravings strike. These options can help satisfy hunger and provide a source of protein and healthy fats while keeping caloric intake manageable.

Finding ideal methods will require some experimentation. It's good to tune into what your body wants while working to find a balance that supports your goals and is sustainable.

The Relationship Between Stress and Food Cravings

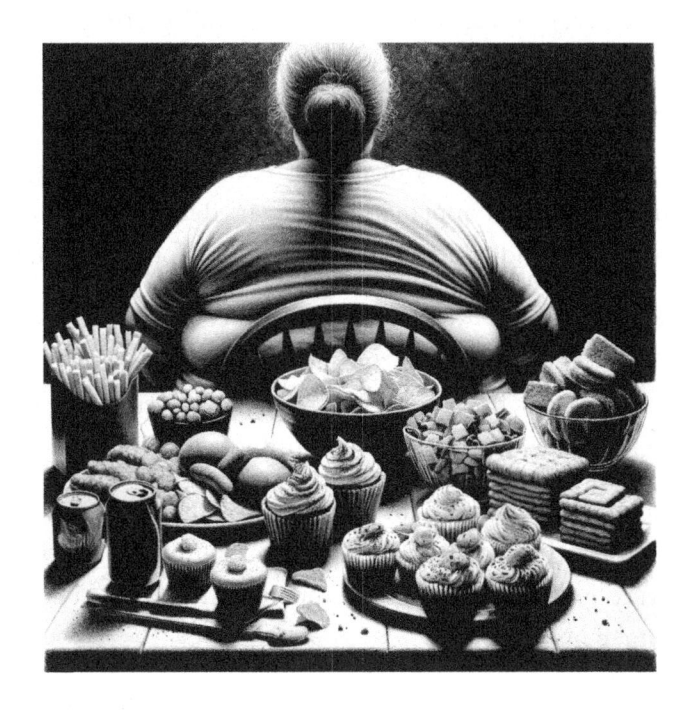

According to researchers at the Garvan Neuroscience Institute (2023), stress plays a vital role in cravings. When you're feeling emotionally stressed, experiencing sleep deprivation, or dealing with an illness, you tend to turn to comfort foods that are high in fat, sugar, and calories.

These low-nutrient foods provide temporary relief and pleasure, helping you cope with stress. However, they lead to weight gain. Further, your body will struggle to release weight if you're stressed, regardless of the cause.

You'll find it easier to achieve goals as you uncover the root causes of stress-related cravings and break those dysfunctional ties. Address the underlying reasons why you crave certain foods and work on changing your relationship with them.

Doing so may involve one or all of the following:

- Talking to a counselor.
- Practicing meditation.
- Forgiving others and yourself.
- Finding alternative outlets for stress, such as exercise, sports, music, or reading.

Lack of sleep can promote stress, increase hunger, and make it more challenging for your body to burn fat during your fasting window. Establish a regular sleep routine and prioritize quality slumber.

Good sleep hygiene helps to regulate hormones, promotes tissue healing and restoration, and improves cognition. All of these benefits can help you to move beyond a plateau.

PLATEAUS AND PROGRESS STALLS

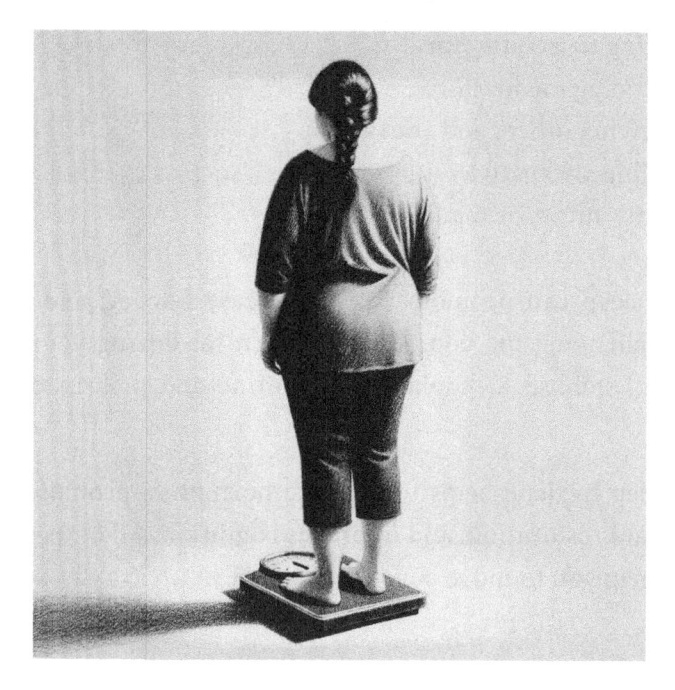

Intermittent fasting can be an effective way to manage weight and improve your health overall. However, it's common to experience stalls in your progress. Let's look at some reasons for plateaus and discuss strategies for overcoming them.

Common Causes of Plateaus

Lack of Consistency

Plateaus can occur when you're not consistently following a fasting schedule. It's vital to adhere to your eating and non-eating windows to maintain the metabolic benefits of intermittent fasting; skipping fasting days can hinder progress.

Keep your fasting window between 14 and 18 hours instead of completely missing it for one or more days.

If traveling or some other event makes it impossible to fast, make up for the 'miss' on the other days. For example, you could get back on track with a 5:2 fast before resuming your usual TRE regimen.

Calorie Intake

When on a fasting plan, you're not restricted in terms of your calorie intake, but it's still necessary to be in a calorie deficit for weight loss. If you consume too many calories during your eating window, it can lead to a plateau. Keep track of your food intake and ensure it aligns with your weight loss goals.

Unhealthy Food Choices

The quality of the food that you eat matters. If you're not making nutritious choices during your eating window, it can hinder your progress. Opt for whole, unprocessed foods and a balanced diet with lean proteins, healthy fats, vegetables, and whole grains. Avoid sugary and high-calorie foods.

12 Strategies for Overcoming Stalls and Plateaus

Here, I've compiled some tips to help you break through a weight loss stall, get things moving again, and regain momentum on your intermittent fasting journey.

- **Preplan for success:** Anticipate potential challenges and be prepared. Before starting your fasting period, make sure you have a good supply of healthy, low glycemic, and anti-inflammatory foods available. This winning strategy will help you to avoid reaching for unhealthy options when hunger strikes.
- **Practice intelligent grocery shopping:** Plan your meals in advance and create a grocery list focusing on nutritious

foods. Stick to your list! If you have wholesome options at home, you'll be more likely to stay on track during your eating window.
- **Preselect menu items:** If you're going out to eat, take the time to review the menu beforehand. Identify which foods meet your macro needs and stay within your caloric goals.

For example, I love a good steak bowl with one spoonful of brown rice, beans, lettuce, cheese, and sauteed vegetables. I can get two meals out of a single bowl without exceeding my macros and daily calorie count. My friend gets two spoons of rice and squeezes three meals out of a bowl!

- **Lean on your support group:** Surround yourself with a good network of friends, family, or fellow fasting fanatics. Share your progress, challenges, and goals with them. They can provide encouragement and helpful tips based on their own experiences.
- **Stick to your macros:** I keep harping on this because it's one of the simplest things you can do to ensure success. If you're following a specific macronutrient ratio or diet plan, such as low-carb or keto, adhere to it during your eating window. Consistency is key!

Additionally, be patient and give your body time to adjust. Plateaus are common and temporary. Trust the process and stay committed to your goals.

- **Focus on non-scale victories:** Celebrate accomplishments beyond the numbers on the scale. Recognize improvements like fitting into smaller-sized clothes, increased energy levels, better lab results, or greater endurance during physical activities. These achievements

indicate positive changes in your body, even if the scale doesn't show significant progress.
- **Manage stress:** When you're constantly stressed, worried, or ill, your body won't release any unwanted weight. Take some time to nourish your mental health to make it easier for your body to lose weight.

Engage in practices that assist you in managing states of worry. These could include exercise, prayer or meditation, and participating in activities you enjoy.

- **Prioritize sleep:** Adequate slumber is crucial for hormonal balance and overall well-being. Use your smartwatch or fitness tracker to monitor your sleep patterns, and keep working on stress reduction until the hours in deep sleep are between one and a half and two hours per night.
- **Strategically time your meals:** Allow your body to burn fat during the night by having your last meal at least 2–3 hours or more before bedtime. Focus on consuming most calories earlier in the day and opt for lighter meals or a protein shake in the evening.
- **Choose nutrient-dense foods:** Foods rich in fiber and protein provide satiety and support weight loss efforts. Avoid sugary or unhealthy foods, even if their calorie counts are similar to healthier options because they can hinder progress.
- **Recognize the role of muscle building:** Healthy muscle bulk contributes to weight loss, even if the scale doesn't change significantly. Your body will trim down as you engage in targeted exercises to tone or increase muscle mass.

Remember that muscle weighs more than fat; don't be shocked if the number on the scale goes up initially.

- **Practice patience and allow for adaptation:** Give your body time to get used to the changes. The longer you adhere to your intermittent fasting plan, the more your body will adapt to lower hunger levels, fat stores, and a new sense of satiety. Be patient, stay consistent, and trust the process.

With all the nuggets you learned from this chapter, you can confidently overcome barriers to progress with intermittent fasting. It's common to hit a plateau, but your fasting journey doesn't need to end there.

Since this book is geared toward women over 50, it's important to talk about 'the change' that we all have gone through. In the next chapter, we'll explore how menopause can affect hormonal balance and metabolism and how intermittent fasting can help.

MAKE A DIFFERENCE WITH YOUR REVIEW

UNLOCK THE POWER OF INTERMITTENT FASTING

"Helping one person might not change the whole world, but it could change the world for one person."

— ANONYMOUS

Did you know that people who generously give of themselves, expecting nothing in return, often live more prosperous and joyful lives? That's not just about money—it's about happiness, fulfillment, and even longevity. Let's take this opportunity to spread a little joy together.

I have a small favor to ask of you...

Would you help a stranger, even if you didn't get a thank you?

Imagine someone like you or perhaps how you were not too long ago. They're over 50, eager to make a positive change in their life, looking for guidance but unsure where to start.

My goal is to share the wonders of intermittent fasting with everyone. Everything I do is driven by this passion. But to truly make a difference, I need to reach... well, everyone.

And this is where you come in. People tend to judge a book by its cover (and what others say about it). Please share your thoughts on this book by leaving a review.

It doesn't cost a penny and takes less than a minute, but the impact? It could be life-changing! Your review might help...

...another woman feel confident and healthy again.
...someone's friend, mom, or grandma discover the joy of feeling good in their body.
...a person just like you feel connected and supported.
...a dreamer achieve their health and weight loss goals.
...transform a life.

Feeling that 'feel good' vibe and ready to make a difference? It's simple and quick to leave a review.

Just scan the QR code below to share your thoughts:

If you're excited about making a positive impact on another person's life, even if you'll never meet them, then you are my kind of person. Welcome to the club!

I can't wait to help you reach your health and wellness goals more effectively and enjoyably than you ever imagined. You're going to love the benefits, tips, and strategies waiting for you in the chapters ahead.

Thank you from the deepest part of my heart. Let's get back to our journey to health and happiness!

- Your biggest cheerleader, Maxine

PS - Here's a little secret: Sharing is caring. If you believe this book can help another woman over 50, don't hesitate to pass it on.

UNDERSTAND THE IMPACT OF MENOPAUSE ON HORMONES

Every woman who has entered the menopausal period understands what I can attest from personal experience: It can be brutal! We have 'the pause' coming at us from every angle: hot flashes, mental fog, emotional swings, weight gain, and a host of other issues; it's a lot!

I'm in the same situation as you and find it beneficial to understand what's happening, why it's happening, and how to handle the changes. It's also helpful to see the positive impact that intermittent fasting can have on the menopause experience.

HORMONAL CHANGES IN WOMEN OVER 50

Menopause marks a natural, programmed halt in ovarian function, which signals the end of a woman's menstrual cycle. It typically happens between 45 and 55 years of age.

However, chromosomal abnormality or an autoimmune disease may cause premature menopause, which occurs when women under the age of 40 lose ovarian function. Surgery or other medical treatments also have the potential to cause early menopause, depending on whether or not the ovaries are present.

Menopause isn't just a matter of cessation in the menstrual cycle. Women who have had reproductive organ surgery or used hormonal contraception experience an end to their periods before the onset of menopause.

As long as the ovaries are still present, the non-menopausal woman will continue to have the ability to produce eggs and estrogen and menstruate. These abilities cease with menopause, as evidenced by 12 consecutive months of no menstrual bleeding.

Menopause is affected by factors such as your well-being, past reproductive experiences, general lifestyle, and environmental shifts. Good premenopausal self-care ensures a healthy transition and the highest quality of life.

If not approached correctly, hormonal changes during menopause can cause disruptions in your social, psychological, emotional, and physical health. Women in their 20s, 30s, and 40s have the best opportunity to promote health and well-being, ensuring easy adjustment to life in their 50s.

Experiences vary from person to person. How you feel during and after the menopausal transition will likely differ from someone else's experience. Some women have few to no symptoms; others may have severe changes that impact their ability to perform everyday tasks.

Menopause-related symptoms include

- nocturnal sweats and hot flashes. These flashes are abrupt feelings of heat in the face, neck, and chest. Skin redness, sweating, racing heartbeat, and intense discomfort in the

body typically follow hot flashes and persist for several minutes.
- alterations to the consistency of the menstrual cycle and flow that lead to the termination of periods.
- vaginal dryness, discomfort during sex, and reduced control over urination.
- difficulty falling asleep.
- shifting emotions, including bouts of sadness or worry.

Estrogen is responsible for the cardioprotective advantage that women have over men when it comes to heart and vascular disease. This protection progressively vanishes after menopause. A woman's risk for osteopenia, osteoporosis, and bone fractures will increase significantly.

The pelvic support structures may also become weaker because of the transition. A weak pelvic floor increases the risk of organ prolapse, where the uterus, bladder, or both can start to move into the vagina. Resulting symptoms include pain and urinary incontinence due to the increased pressure on the bladder.

Discuss any symptoms or concerns that you experience with your healthcare provider. A comprehensive evaluation should consider medical history, values, and preferences to identify potential treatment options, including hormonal and non-hormonal therapies.

Some women experience vaginal bleeding after menopause. Most of the time, the cause is benign or non-cancerous. Sometimes, it can occur due to preexisting endometriosis, cysts, or polyps. Vaginal dryness can also cause postmenopausal bleeding.

In a small percentage of women over 50, vaginal bleeding may indicate a more worrisome problem such as cancer. The only way to know is to get a thorough gynecologic exam as soon as possible.

Early intervention will increase the chances for a speedy diagnosis and the best treatment options and outcomes.

Intermittent Fasting and Hormone Balance

Estrogen levels become unpredictable during menopause before dropping significantly once the transition is complete. Changes associated with cortisol, thyroid hormones, serotonin, and sex hormones are also evident during menopause. These shifts bring on some of the signs and symptoms that annoy and frustrate us day and night.

During menopause, your insulin sensitivity may decrease, making it harder for your body to process refined sugars and carbohydrates. This condition is called insulin resistance, which can increase your risk of accumulating fat. Naturally, this will lead to weight gain.

It's also possible that muscle mass will decrease as fat deposits increase, which will reduce the amount of metabolically active tissue available to burn calories. If this happens, maintaining a healthy weight becomes more challenging.

Intermittent fasting may help women over 50 who frequently encounter unwelcome fluctuations in their blood sugar, body fat, and even blood lipid levels. The following points highlight the benefits of fasting during and post-menopause (WebMD, 2021a):

- **Improved insulin sensitivity:** Insensitivity develops because estrogen, essential to moving glucose into cells, is reduced. Intermittent fasting increases insulin sensitivity by giving the body more time to move glucose out of the bloodstream.

Fat becomes the primary fuel source after 12 hours of fasting, and the body becomes more sensitive and responsive to insulin.

- **Increased human growth hormone:** Intermittent fasting naturally increases HGH, a crucial hormone for metabolism and glucose regulation. HGH enhances insulin sensitivity.
- **Improved mental health:** The emotional roller coaster accompanying menopause can stabilize through fasting. Mental wellness can also improve as fasting reduces stress and boosts self-esteem.

Despite all of the benefits just mentioned, intermittent fasting can sometimes cause disruptions that may aggravate menopause symptoms. This possibility underscores the importance of easing into fasting.

You are unique, and it may take you more time to find a comfortable rhythm than others. Start with a 12:12 or 14:10 version for three to four weeks to see how it affects you before trying a more demanding interval.

Know your body, and discuss any concerns with your healthcare provider. Try not to rely on self-diagnosis or 'Dr. Google'.

MENOPAUSE AND THE RISK OF OSTEOPOROSIS

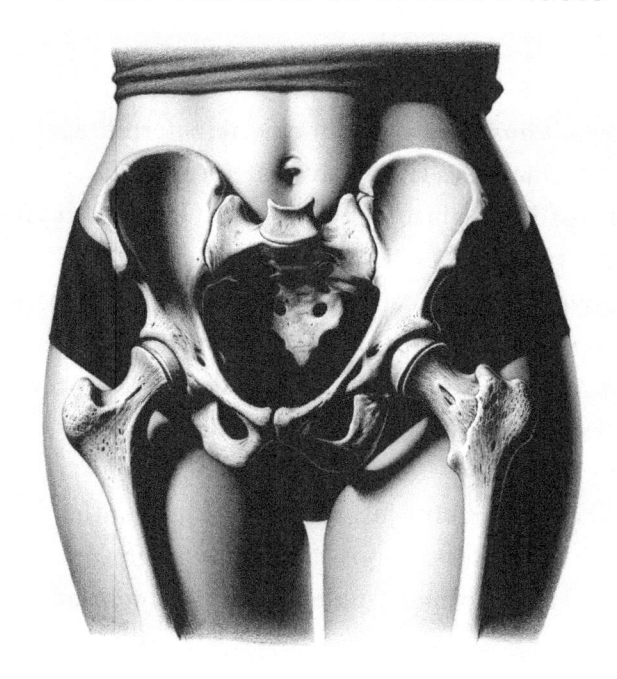

As we age, calcium is leeched from the bones and moved into the circulation to maintain normal blood levels. This change causes low bone mass and bone tissue degeneration, which are signs of osteoporosis. Both of these conditions increase bone fragility and fracture risk.

Statistics have it that 50% of women over 50 will suffer at least one fracture throughout their lifetime, mainly because of poor bone health (Bolster, 2023). The most common areas for fragility fractures are the spine, wrists, and hips.

Complete or partial bone breaks may cause discomfort, restrict activity, undermine self-confidence, and lower the quality of life. Complications of fractures can lead to social isolation and associated depression.

Premature menopause in women can also increase the risks for osteoporosis, whether brought on naturally or by medical procedures, surgery, chemotherapy, malnutrition, or other means. Conditions such as anorexia can lead to a reduction in estrogen and bone density, significantly increasing fracture risk.

Obesity is a risk factor that indirectly impacts bone strength because of the excessive physical stress associated with carrying extra weight. Also, fatty tissue is less protective and supportive of health than skeletal muscle.

Inflammatory changes often accompany excess fat or adipose tissue, which disrupts bone growth and strength. However, a very low body mass index or weight-to-height ratio might also increase fracture risk as there is less tissue to cushion the force of a fall.

Social habits can predispose women to poor bone density. As a matter of fact, smoking harms the ovaries and bones. Further, smoking is associated with an increased risk of chronic health problems, many different cancers - not just lung cancer - and death. Even alcohol can disrupt normal bone formation and increase the risk of osteoporosis.

Take heart; you can reduce all of the previously discussed risks by changing your lifestyle. You owe it to yourself to be as healthy as possible in and after menopause.

ASSESSING AND REDUCING FRACTURE RISK

Ideally, women should start bone density checks at age 65, using a specific type of X-ray called a DEXA scan. Talk to your healthcare provider about when you should start, as you may have unique health circumstances or a family history that warrants earlier testing.

Strategies for Supporting Bone and Muscle Health

Bone tissue is constantly degrading and rebuilding. As we age, the rate of breakdown exceeds replacement. This change results in porous bones that are sluggish; they don't regrow fast enough to prevent brittleness and breaking.

The good news is that we can incorporate lifestyle changes, even now, that can slow or reverse bone loss. There are also things that we can do to maintain muscle mass, which is protective against osteoporosis. Let's discuss some of them now.

Exercise Every Day

Workouts involving impact and resistance to build muscle can increase bone strength, lowering the chance of injury. When done correctly, these exercises may also help manage pain and discomfort from vertebral fractures.

Impact workouts include jogging, stair climbing, tennis, aerobics, and anything else that makes your feet stomp with force. As a result of the force, your bones will become stronger and denser in the presence of adequate dietary calcium.

Low-impact exercises like walking and using an elliptical machine are also excellent options if you find high-impact exercises hard on your joints. Water aerobics is an alternative low-force exercise that can help strengthen bones and muscles.

Weightlifting and workouts with resistance bands, dumbbells, or your body weight will condition and strengthen muscles. Yoga, chair exercises, and tai chi can also help.

If finding the time to exercise is challenging, opt for high-intensity interval training (HIIT) or similar. HIIT exercises allow you to get away with just seven to 10 minutes of exercise alone, plus a brief warming and cooling period.

Adopt a Diet High in Calcium

Your body needs calcium for various physiologic processes; if you don't get enough of it from your food, it will come from your bones. This mineral is present in dairy products, fruits like figs and oranges, fish like salmon and sardines, beans, and soy products.

Vegetables like broccoli, Brussels sprouts, kale, and spinach are also calcium-rich. Vitamins D and K help the body and bones absorb calcium, so don't forget them.

If you are on blood thinners, consult your healthcare provider before increasing your dark greens and vitamin K intake. The blood thinner was likely initiated to be consistent with your previous state of health. A dietary increase in vitamin K intake can interact with your blood thinner and put you at risk for clotting or bleeding problems.

Try to get 1,200 mg of calcium from your diet every day. For example, a breakfast of yogurt and cheese on whole grain bread, a lunch with steamed broccoli, greens, or bok choy, and an early evening smoothie with spinach, kale, and milk would bring your calcium intake up to the required levels.

Ask your healthcare provider if you should take supplements or if you have a condition that calcium supplementation can aggravate. Recall that women over 50 are at a higher risk for heart conditions. Calcium supplementations can increase risks for cardiovascular disease.

Get Adequate Vitamin D

Your body can absorb calcium more efficiently with help from vitamin D. Sunshine is a commonly available source, but if you live in a state like Oregon, you'll need some help. The same holds true for those who live in areas of the country or world with limited opportunities to spend time in the sun.

Vitamin D deficiency is common even in places that get a good amount of sunshine because residents spend a lot of time indoors and out of the heat. As little as 10 to 30 minutes of exposure to the sun most days of the week can help to keep levels normal.

Get your vitamin D levels checked before attempting to take supplements. Lab testing will give an accurate idea of where you stand and how many units you should take daily or weekly.

Limit Sugar and Salt Intake

Excessive sugar and salt (sodium) intake threatens bone density. When you consume either of these substances, your kidneys try to excrete as much as possible to restore balance.

Calcium, an innocent bystander, gets eliminated from the body along with these white, crystalline villains. The inflammatory effect of sugar on the kidneys poses an additional threat because it increases the risk of low bone mineral density more significantly than salt.

Here's a fun fact (Healthline, 2018): Keeping your salt intake well below two grams daily (about one-third of a teaspoon) can improve mood in postmenopausal women. Make every effort to reduce dietary sugar and sodium from all sources, especially processed foods.

HORMONE REPLACEMENT THERAPY (HRT)

The body naturally produces estrogen, progesterone, and testosterone until menopause. Symptoms that we associate with menopause are directly related to the fact that these hormone levels have dropped.

HRT aims to replace some of these hormones to manage or eliminate the uncomfortable and troublesome symptoms. The estrogen, progesterone, and testosterone used in therapeutic preparations are typically plant-based. However, some may be formulated with animal products such as horse urine or gel from cows.

Compounded HRTs, sometimes called bioidentical hormones, are prepared by pharmacists and tailored to an individual's unique prescription. They are formulated to closely resemble the hormones produced by the body's endocrine glands. Depending on the pharmacy, the compound may contain animal products.

Conventionally-produced HRTs are developed in laboratories to address general menopause symptoms. These medicines are not custom-made for individuals. Some are bioidentical, and not all contain animal products.

The Food and Drug Administration (FDA) approves lab-derived HRT based on scientific studies showing a degree of effectiveness and safety in the general population. Compounded hormones are not FDA-approved as they are not produced or tested in a lab for the general population.

Both FDA-approved and compounded HRT come in various forms, and both types of hormones require a prescription.

In theory, HRT should help to reduce menopause symptoms and restore some of the protective benefits that are lost due to reduced hormone levels. However, there are risks associated with HRT, including clotting disorders, heart disease, breast cancer, and stroke, regardless of the source of the hormones.

An obstetrician, gynecologist, or other healthcare provider with special training in hormone replacement is an excellent resource for more information on this topic. The decision to take HRT or not is individual; seek professional advice and weigh the pros and cons of your unique situation.

SAFEGUARD YOUR HEALTH

The menopausal and postmenopausal periods present opportunities to safeguard your health. You can do this in part by monitoring what you eat and drink.

Limit processed foods, simple carbohydrates, and added sugars, such as those present in white bread, crackers, store-bought snacks, and baked goods. Doing so can help reduce symptoms like hot flashes, weight gain, and poor sleep associated with menopause. In addition, avoid

Caffeine and Alcohol

Hot flashes can be aggravated by caffeine and alcohol in menopausal women. Try giving up caffeine for several months to see if the elimination reduces your symptoms. Consider the fact that many menopausal women who drink have difficulties sleeping because alcohol disturbs sleep (Pacheco and Singh, 2020).

Spicy Food

When going through menopause, try to steer clear of spicy-hot foods. A 2018 Healthline study compared lifestyle characteristics to hot flash frequency in 896 menopausal women from Spain and South America. Women who consumed spicy foods experienced hot flashes more frequently than those who did not.

NAVIGATING MENOPAUSE WITH INTERMITTENT FASTING

If intermittent fasting is done correctly, it can provide benefits that counteract some of the negative changes associated with menopause.

Adopt one or more of the following suggestions for best results:

- Start with a brief fasting window, such as 12:12 or 14:10, and progressively transition to a more stringent method to reduce fasting-related changes in mood.
- Adopt a healthy, balanced diet.
- Drink plenty of water.
- Eat with awareness, pay attention to your body's needs, and, if necessary, shorten your fasting window.
- Take steps to prevent or minimize stress, anxiety, and disordered eating.
- Take advantage of online resources, but don't use them as a substitute for professional advice.
- Join a support group.

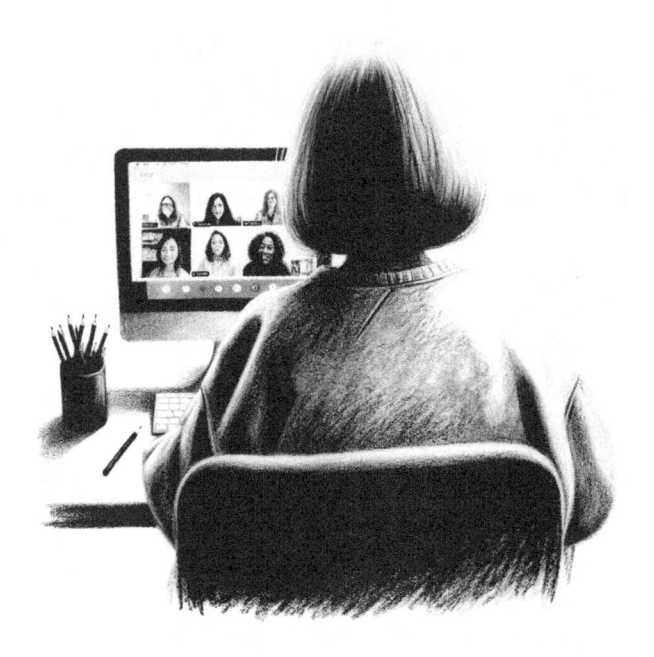

Often, women feel like they have to tackle significant changes like a new fasting journey all alone; that's not true! Solid female relationships are advantageous and may keep you mentally and emotionally healthy as you age.

Sharing your intermittent fasting ups and downs helps to validate feelings as you sort through worries, fears, setbacks, and discomforts.

Five Tips for Promoting Emotional Health During Menopause

Reduced estrogen levels during menopause might trigger additional stressors that can negatively affect your day-to-day life. Weight gain, low self-esteem, osteoporosis, and impending hazards to heart health can all contribute to higher stress.

Women who are going through the menopausal transition may also experience despair and anxiety. Take heart; there is something that you can do to improve your emotional health during this time of change.

In addition to eating well, you can look and feel younger by exercising and caring for your mental health. The following five strategies can help you to handle emotions successfully (Bitsoli, 2022).

Accept the Change

Stress may increase as you struggle with the unpleasant feelings brought on by hormonal changes in your body. Keep your cool and accept menopause as a normal and unavoidable part of life. This shift in mindset is a beneficial coping method that encourages emotional control instead of a feeling of helplessness.

Take Back Your Sexual Life

Time spent between the sheets can be affected by decreased estrogen production and an associated loss of interest in sex. This issue is worth addressing because sexual activity is a proven, effective stress reliever.

During an orgasm, hormones like dopamine and oxytocin are released, making you feel at ease, joyful, and sleepy. Vaginal dryness can be brought on by decreased estrogen production, but lubricants can help. Don't let menopause dictate or ruin your bedroom life.

Exercise Regularly

Physical activity enhances the production of endorphins, which are *happy* hormones. Thus, exercise has a substantial impact on alleviating stress. A decent workout also encourages deeper sleep while the stress chemicals—cortisol and adrenaline—are depleted during workouts.

I've included 12 exercises in the next chapter, and there are many online resources by professionals to choose from.

Become Friends With Sleep

Poor sleep can result from ongoing stress, hot flashes, mood swings, anxiety, and depression. Sleep deficits can hurt your heart, mind, and cognitive abilities. Due to the relationship between sleep and stress, a vicious cycle can result from problems in either area.

After a night of insufficient rest, you'll be exhausted, irritable, moody, and have difficulty concentrating. Each of these symptoms has the potential to negatively impact your work, home, and social experiences.

Getting between seven and nine hours of sleep every day is essential. A regular bedtime and waking schedule might boost your sleep duration. Keep your room quiet, cold, dark, and comfortable. Also, avoid caffeine and stressful situations before bed.

Laugh Often

Look for comedy in daily experiences; it's a simple way to manage worry, ease tension, and lift your spirits. Laughing lowers cortisol levels in the body and raises endorphin levels in the brain. When you laugh, more oxygen enters your lungs, improving circulation and lowering blood pressure.

Finding an enjoyable activity, such as watching humorous videos, scrolling funny memes, or reading a comic book, is good. Pamper yourself often, and spend more time with friends and loved ones.

In the following chapter, we'll dive deeper into how intermittent fasting goes hand-in-hand with exercise. The stress relief that comes with physical activity helps improve mood and makes life much more enjoyable.

HOW FASTING AND EXERCISE WORK TOGETHER

In January 2023, I started being intentional about intermittent fasting to control my weight, which has served me well! However, fasting didn't create lean muscle mass, flatten my abdomen, or strengthen my bones. My floppy arms and belly bore witness to these facts!

It wasn't until I started incorporating exercise that I saw a toner, leaner, curvier figure with less jiggling. My flabby parts were getting rearranged just the way I wanted.

Now, I feel super confident in telling all of you that to achieve the best overall results with intermittent fasting, you should incorporate some form of exercise into your daily or weekly regimen.

Properly scheduling your fasting and workout routines according to your body's ability and health requirements will help you reap the full benefits in comparatively little time. In this chapter, I'll explain how you can do this effectively.

THE SYNERGY OF EXERCISE AND FASTING

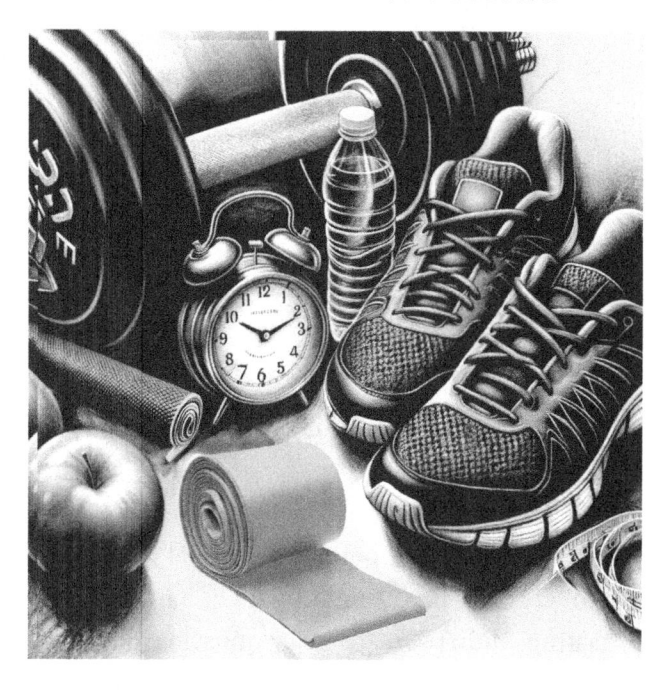

You'll notice your body transforming beautifully between your second and third month of intermittent fasting as clothes begin to fit looser and fat cells reduce in size. Your general and mental health improve fairly early after adopting a fasting plan.

Remember to celebrate these fantastic changes in your body!

However, there are some physical benefits that you may not be able to enjoy by practicing intermittent fasting on its own without supplementary physical activity. Here are a couple worth noting:

- **You won't be able to build muscle mass**: Fasting may lead to changes that result in a body shape you don't necessarily desire. As you just read from my experiences with fasting alone, I was left with a lot of flab!

Exercise helps to tone your muscles and trim fatty areas around the armpits, bra line, and abdomen. Over time, the wrinkles and flabby regions will smooth out and disappear. Be patient! This process can take months.

- **You won't improve bone density or strength**: It is essential to replenish lost bone matter to enhance its density. The stress on bones that occurs with exercising is a great way to get this done!

In light of these factors, incorporate a regular exercise regimen with intermittent fasting to maximize the benefits.

How to Incorporate Exercises Into Your Fasting Routine for Best Results

Find the Ideal Time of the Day to Fast

Try to initiate your fast during the latter hours of the day and overnight. Damjanovic's research (2022) shows fasting during the early morning is less beneficial than skipping a late evening snack or dinner. Starting your fasting window well before bedtime also reduces your chance of eating junk food, which is higher at night than during the day.

Optimize fat burning by exercising just before breaking your fast, if possible. For most people, this means you'll exercise in the morning.

When you exercise in a fasted state, your body will burn fat to fuel your workout. If you break your fast before exercising, the nutrients you consume will be used to fuel your physical activity, and fat will be spared.

Alternatively, pack most of your nutritional intake as early in your day as possible without leaving yourself starved and craving junk food during the evening hours. Have your last meal early enough in the evening to complete digestion before exercising.

For example, you could have a light dinner and start fasting as early as 5 or 6 p.m., exercise two to three hours later, and then get to bed around 10-10:30 p.m. in a fasting state. Post-workout, drink water with or without fresh lemon slices, apple cider vinegar, or herbal teas to ensure good hydration.

If you work overnight hours, you'll need to adjust fasting and exercise times to achieve the desired results. See Chapter 3 for tips on finding an ideal fasting interval to complement your work schedule.

Incorporate Resistance in Your Workouts

Exercises such as push-ups, sit-ups, leg raises, and squats only require pushing your weight within a free physical space. These bodyweight exercises provide enough resistance to preserve your muscle mass while getting rid of excess body fat, helping you to attain a slim body shape.

Another benefit of bodyweight exercises is that they cost you nothing, require no equipment, and you can do them anywhere.

Prepare Your Mind

Use online resources to review a few body-weight exercises for arms, trunk, back, and legs before diving into a routine. Select the ones you feel most comfortable trying without hurting yourself. Do them consistently over one to two weeks to get a feel of which to incorporate into your workout routine.

A general convention is to exercise the upper body areas, including the shoulder, arm, and hand muscles, along with your abdominal and core muscles one day. On alternating days, exercise the back muscles, the buttocks, hips, thighs, legs, and feet.

12 Strength and Conditioning Exercises

The following exercises are easy and safe to do and a good option for those who feel apprehensive about exercising due to inexperience, physical ailments, or other limitations. If you want a more challenging regimen, check out the myriad online resources with videos you can follow.

Physical and occupational therapists and other healthcare professionals post some of the best workout routines online. Look for videos that show modifications for beginners, as those adaptations will help to prevent injuries.

Start slow and focus more on form than repetitions. Once you can do the exercises correctly, aim to complete five to ten repetitions (a set), followed by a 30 to 60-second rest period. Do three sets of each exercise before moving on to another.

You can practice

1. Seated chest squeezes: Begin this exercise by sitting upright with a straightened back. This erect position helps tighten your abdominal and core muscles to support your back.

Start with elbows bent and hands touching in the prayer position. Lower the forearms until both are parallel to the ground. Push the palms together for about three seconds, then relax.

If done correctly, you should feel your wrist muscles stretching and your chest muscles tightening. Repeat this motion three times to complete a set, shake out your arms, and continue to perform the exercise until you have finished three sets.

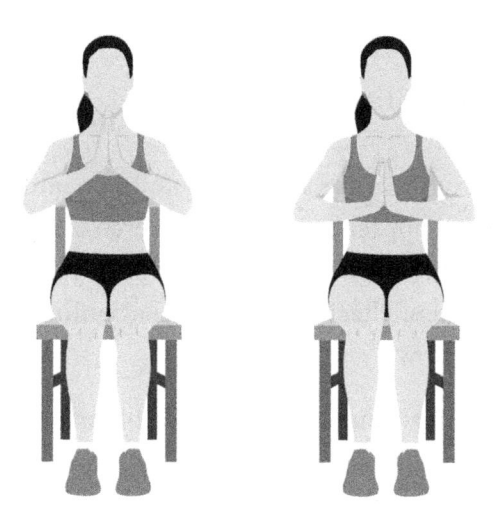

2. Standing shoulder retractions with a resistance band: Tighten your abdominal and core muscles to support your back while standing straight. Hold a long resistance band at chest height with both hands and extend your elbows.

Pull both shoulders back simultaneously as the arms move off to the side and the resistance band moves toward your body. Return to the starting position to complete a repetition.

You'll feel this exercise working the muscles in your mid-back and stretching your chest and shoulder muscles.

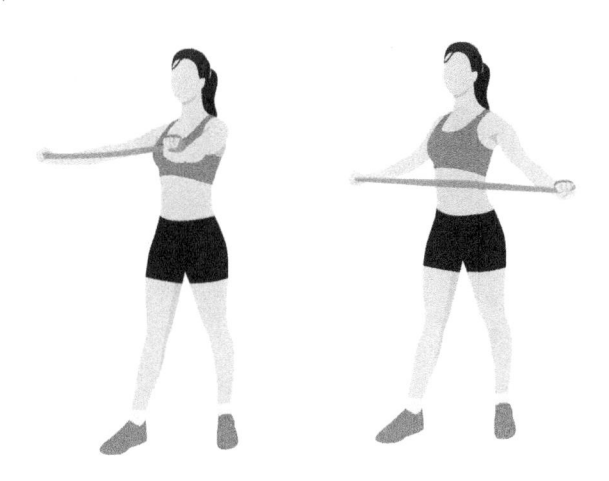

3. Standing chest presses: Stand arm's length away from a wall with your back comfortably straight; keep your feet flat or go up on your toes. Put both palms against the wall, shoulder width apart, at shoulder height. Start with the elbows extended but not locked.

Slowly bend your elbows and lean in until your nose almost touches the wall. Keep the elbows at no more than a 45-degree angle to your body, and don't let them touch your torso. Push away from the wall to complete a repetition.

You'll feel this wall push-up exercise mostly in your chest, shoulder, and arms.

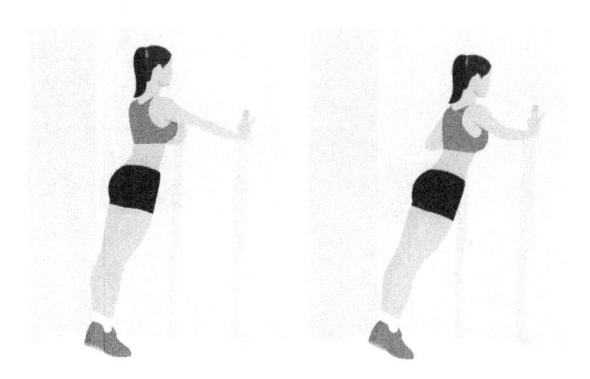

4. Seated knee lifts: Sit comfortably with your back upright, abdominal and core muscles squeezed, and feet flat. Slowly flex at your hip by lifting one leg up to a comfortable height, then return your foot to the ground. Repeat this motion with the other hip.

To intensify the workout, try the following: Hold your leg in the flexed position up to a count of seven, then slowly let it back down. Make the same motion with the other leg. This exercise will give your hip area an intense workout.

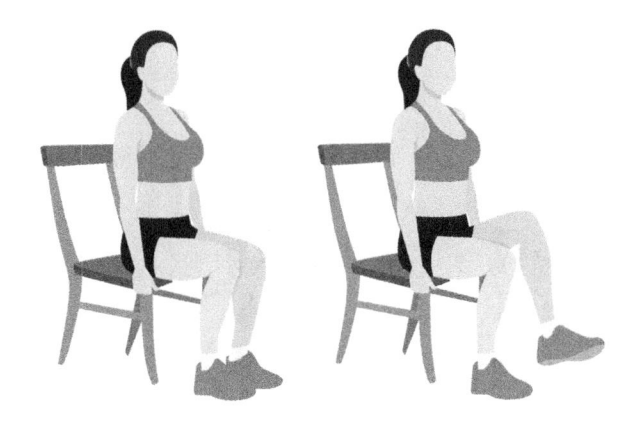

5. Seated knee extensions: Keep your back upright, your abdominal and core muscles squeezed, and your feet flat. Slowly straighten one knee as much as possible, then flex it back so your foot returns to the ground. Repeat this motion with the other knee.

Try to do this exercise in three sets as described above, or hold your extended leg position up to a count of seven for a more intense workout, then slowly let it back down. Repeat the same procedure with the other leg.

This exercise will leave your thigh muscles feeling like they went to work!

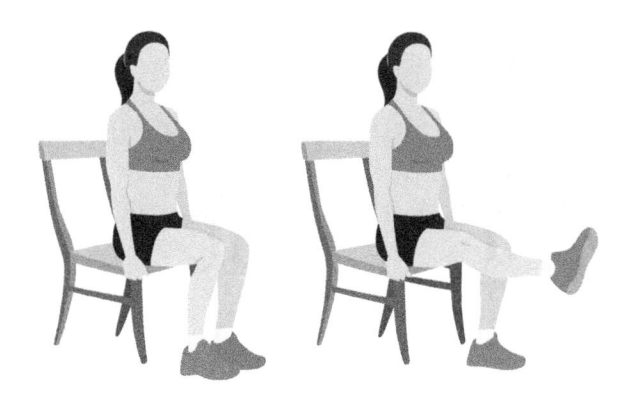

6. Standing heel raises: Start by standing in a semi-squatting position with a wide stance, feet flat and mainly pointing forward, and knees pointing slightly outward. Squeeze your abdominal and core muscles and rest both palms on the front of your upper thighs to maintain the position.

Have a sturdy chair close behind you in case of difficulty holding your balance. Alternatively, do this exercise while seated.

Raise one heel as high as possible, then lower it and repeat on the other side to complete a repetition. Aim for three repetitions per set to start. To intensify this exercise, increase the number of repetitions or raise both heels simultaneously.

Ease into the motions gently, as the muscles in your foot may try to cramp. If that happens, stop the heel raises and give yourself a foot massage. Next time, try warming and massaging the foot before performing this exercise.

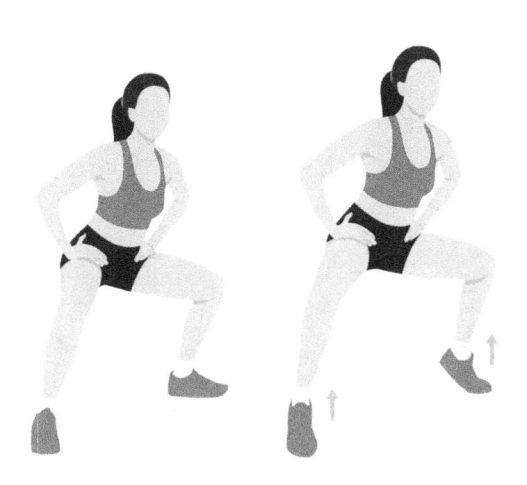

7. Standing leg raises: Stand on one leg while keeping your back straight; stay close to a table or countertop that you can hold for additional support if needed. Squeeze your abdominal and butt muscles as you raise your other straightened leg to cross over the stabilizing foot. This motion will engage the muscles of your inner thigh.

Next, swing the same leg up and out to the side as high as you can comfortably go without straining yourself. This motion will engage the muscles of your outer thigh.

Return the foot to the floor to complete a repetition. Start with only two or three repetitions for a set, then switch sides and repeat. Take your time!

This exercise is excellent for tightening the hip and buttock muscles. However, if you don't pace yourself, it may leave you with aches and regrets! As your abdomen, hip, and core muscles become stronger, you'll find it easier to increase repetitions.

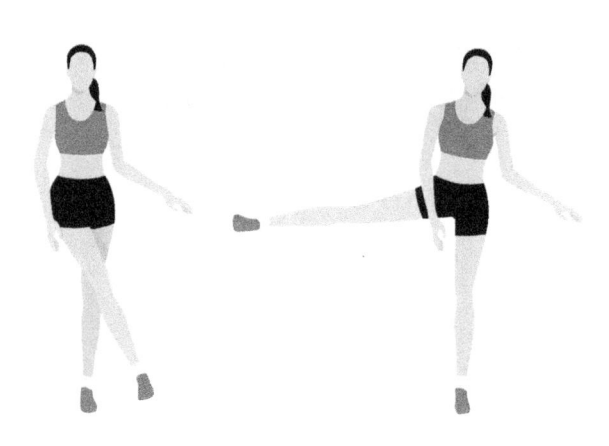

8. Seated torso twists: Keep your feet on the ground while sitting up straight. Fold your arms across your chest and rotate your trunk slowly and carefully to one side, back to neutral, and then rotate to the other side. Stretch your torso as much as possible while keeping the exercise comfortable and pain-free.

You may hear some crackling sounds as you do this exercise; it's just the sound of gas in your spine joints and is of no concern unless you experience pain simultaneously. If that happens, stop this exercise immediately and visit your chiropractor or healthcare provider for an evaluation.

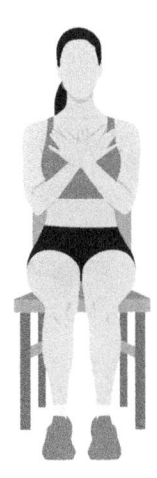

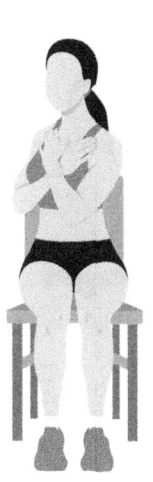

9. Seated side bends: Tighten your abdominal muscles while keeping your back straight and your feet flat. Raise one arm overhead while slowly and gently bending to the side of the unraised arm. Return to the upright position, then repeat the motion three to five more times to complete a set.

Take a 60-second rest, then perform the same exercise on the opposite side.

Hold each bending position for up to 10 seconds to increase exercise intensity. Don't be surprised if your sides look more trim after a few weeks of doing this routine.

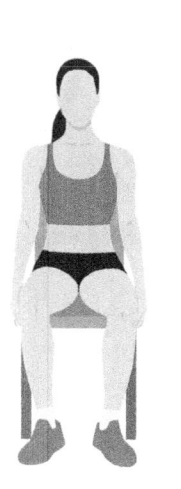

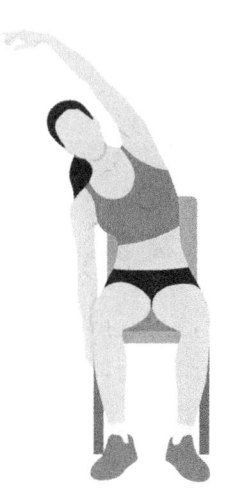

10. Chair squats: Take a position as if you are about to sit on a sturdy seat, with hands close to or slightly touching the chair to support and prevent falling. Position your feet shoulder-width apart and facing forward, with knees slightly angled outward.

Next, sit down carefully then stand back up to complete a repetition. Aim for three to five repetitions per set to start.

You can increase exercise intensity by holding and maintaining your squat position for about five seconds without touching your butt to the seat. To prevent injury, ensure your knees do not extend past the tip of your toes.

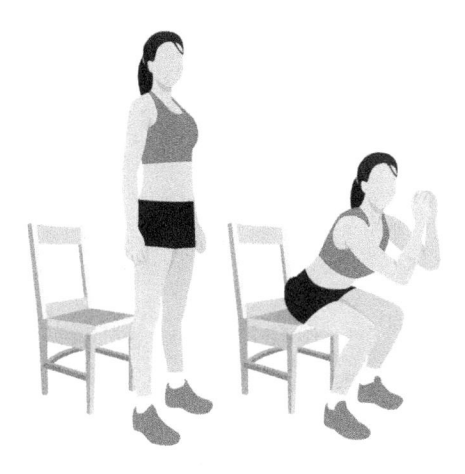

11. Laying chest presses: Start with two small hand weights of equal mass (or a couple of 12-ounce cans from your pantry). Lay down on a firm pillow, a bosu ball (as shown in the illustration), or a yoga mat. Bend your knees so that both feet are planted on the ground.

Take a weight in each hand, then extend your arms without making them completely straight. Elevate your arms so the weights are in front of you at the level of your chest, and your thumbs are touching.

Slowly move the weights down and toward the chest along an imaginary arc until they are shoulder-width apart but still at chest level. As the elbows bend, the back of each upper arm and elbow should move in line with the sides of your torso without touching the pillow, bosu ball, or ground.

Next, move the weights back up to the starting position to complete a repetition. Aim for three sets of up to 10 repetitions with 60 seconds of rest between sets. This particular exercise can also be performed while in a seated position.

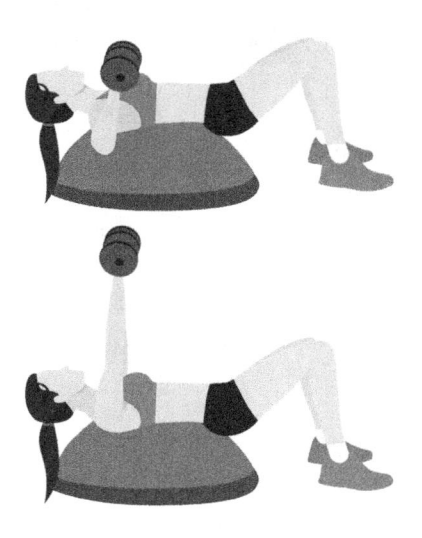

12. Seated alphabet toner: You'll get a good hip and abdominal workout and a toned lower body in time by performing this exercise seated, as shown. Keep your back straight and abdomen tight as you flex at the hip to form letters of the alphabet with one leg. Support your weight with the other foot flat on the ground.

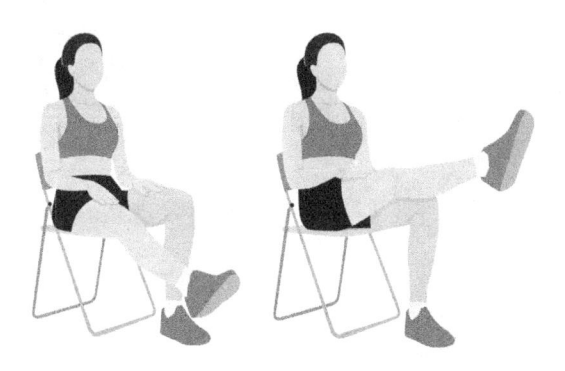

Try doing this exercise from a standing position to help improve balance and proprioception—your awareness of your body's position in its surroundings. Stand on one leg while using the other to form the letters of the alphabet in the air.

The bigger the letters, the more intense the workout. However, it's better for your body and brain if you move your leg through only a few letters with proper form and technique than to rush the process just to get through more letters of the alphabet.

The standing leg keeps you balanced and coordinated by sending feedback information to your brain and responding to commands from the brain. You may be wobbly when you first start this exercise, but keep at it! Your balance will noticeably improve within two to three months.

Intensify Your Workout

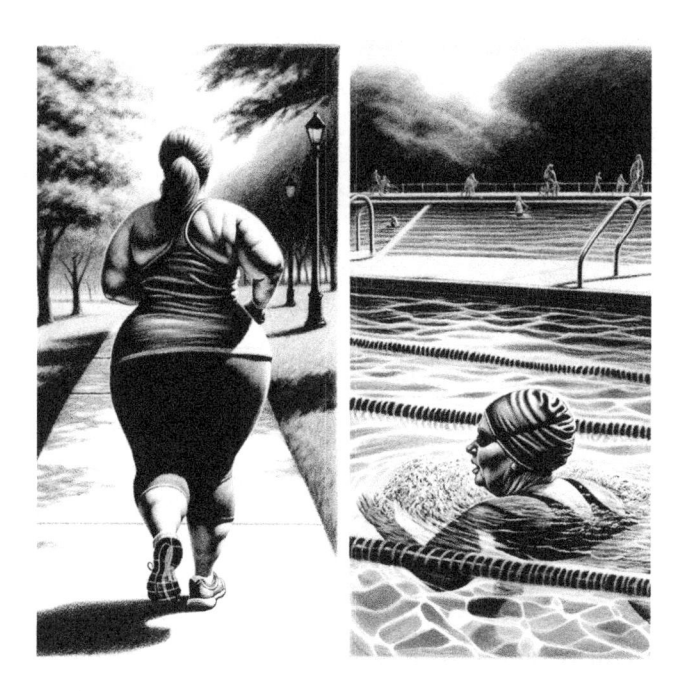

Jogging

Consider jogging a few times weekly to complement your strength and conditioning exercises. Doing so can help you eliminate excess fat and maintain a lean body.

Studies show you can significantly shed excess body fat by about 20% when you exercise on an empty stomach (Zouhal et al., 2020). Jogging while in your fasting window can also help you overcome nausea, a common experience for older women who exercise soon after eating.

Start with a slow, gentle jog, and pace yourself. Listen to your body when it's telling you to stop.

Swimming

Pool time can add variety to your workout routine. Swimming develops and strengthens your hand, shoulder, leg, and back muscles and helps build your abs. Swimming also improves your coordination and balance significantly.

If you're not a swimmer, walking the pool length in the shallow end can help you maximize fat burning. Keep water and a healthy shake on hand for quick recovery and replenishment after exercising.

How to Structure Workout Routines Around Fasting Schedules

Your workout routine should not interfere with your fasting schedule or leave you feeling wiped out. Take steps to optimize your energy reserves while making the most of your exercise sessions. Use the following tips to achieve the best results:

- **Exercise heading into your fasting time:** For the first one to three hours after a full or heavy meal, your body is busy digesting your food. Most of your available blood flow will be focused on the gut. Anything more than a brief walk post-meal can lead to an upset stomach and indigestion.

  Hold off exercising until two to three hours after eating, but close to the start of your fasting time to avoid interfering with this process. Plan to do a more intense workout if your last meal was heavy. Give a light snack about 30 minutes to an hour to move through your digestive tract before exercising.

- **Try to maintain moderate workout sessions:** If you're toward the middle or ending of your fasting window and need to exercise, keep your activity mild to moderate. Check your breathing rate to determine the relative intensity of your workout so you can adjust accordingly. Moderate-intensity exercise should allow you to conversate without any difficulty breathing.

Have water and a protein source on hand for post-exercise recovery. A quick snack can provide much-needed energy if you timed your exercise to coincide with ending your fast.

- **Consume meals that have high protein content:** Whether you exercise before, during, or after fasting, a diet with adequate protein intake helps repair and grow muscles. Increase your intake as needed to account for your level of physical activity and usual daily needs.

According to Fetters of the Academy of Nutrition and Dietetics, one protein snack every four hours is recommended for adequate muscle repair and tissue growth (2015). This won't be possible with a 6-hour eating window, but it is achievable with a 12:12, 14:10, and 16:8 fast.

FASTING AND MUSCLE PRESERVATION

Your body's balance between anabolism and catabolism determines your net muscle mass. Anabolism relates to building muscles, while catabolism is the deconstruction of muscle protein to obtain energy.

Whenever you deplete glucose and stored glycogen, your body will resort to gluconeogenesis, using fat and muscle protein as building blocks to make more glucose. The goal is to prevent any loss of muscle. Remember our mantra from Chapter 1? Spare the muscles; burn the fat!

A diet with adequate protein and moderate amounts of healthy fats and carbohydrates will help prevent muscle catabolism while revitalizing your energy. Don't go for prolonged periods without eating anything, especially if you have an underlying medical condition.

As you've discovered, incorporating exercise into your intermittent fasting routine can help you achieve a leaner and curvier body and gain the energy and confidence to keep up with your work and leisure demands. Physical limitations don't have to preclude exercising. Many sitting exercises and other workout modifications can help you achieve fitness goals.

Intermittent fasting also plays a significant role in helping you to think clearly and develop a sharper mind. We'll discuss this benefit further in the next chapter.

NOURISH YOUR MIND

When I started my intermittent fasting journey, I had one goal in mind: to give my stomach the time it needed to heal and reduce irritable bowel syndrome (IBS) symptoms. It was an absolute bonus to discover that fasting is one of the reasons why my mind is as sharp now as it was three decades ago.

Back then, my brain seemed to fire on all cylinders every single day. I was full of energy and seemed to squeeze 36 hours of activity into 24 hours without missing a beat! I never imagined that I could regain that same energy and productivity with fasting.

The focus and mental clarity I experience now allows me to accomplish so much from 5 a.m. to 10 p.m., and I still have steam left over! I'm pushing 60, and just this past week, I successfully pulled an all-nighter to meet a deadline.

My productivity and concentration throughout my eight-hour workday and for another eight hours afterward did not diminish, not even for a minute! Without a doubt, prayer, fasting, and a healthy diet contributed to my mental and physical stamina.

Intermittent fasting is a scientifically proven practice that helps to reduce the impacts of several cognitive conditions like Alzheimer's and Parkinson's disease, autism spectrum disorder, ischemic stroke, anxiety, and depression. Fasting decongests your mind, which enables you to make better decisions; it also improves overall performance.

In addition to fasting, specific nutrients decelerate or slow cognitive decline. Foods such as citrus fruits, strawberries, salmon, tuna, and many others containing vitamins B and E are very protective of brain function.

The extent to which intermittent fasting impacts your mind depends on your diet's specific nutrient content and caloric value. It's also affected by your personal fasting schedule and patterns.

The ball is in your court, ladies! It's up to you to make the most of your fasting routine; this chapter will guide that process.

THE IMPACT OF FASTING ON BRAIN FUNCTION

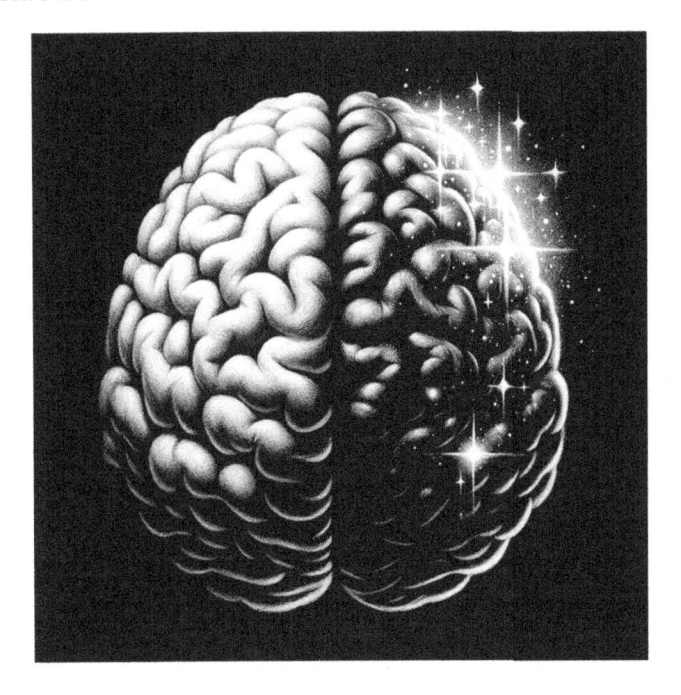

According to Johns Hopkins researchers (2021), the impact of intermittent fasting on your brain primarily results from how and when you eat. The benefits are not just a reflection of the type of food you consume.

Generally, brain function is optimized when the fluidity of your neurons (neuroplasticity) increases; fasting enhances this phenomenon.

Neuroplasticity is synonymous with adaptability; it's how neurons respond to and compensate for challenges that the brain encounters. In short, neuroplasticity improves your brain's resistance to disease and injury.

Intermittent Fasting, Cognitive Function, and Brain Health

The hormonal imbalances that accompany the onset of menopause trigger anxiety, memory lapses, low mood, depression, and irritability. Intermittent fasting

- **Helps you to get rid of excess body fat:** Obesity is associated with depression, low self-esteem, fear of going out, and panic disorder. As the benefits of fasting become physically apparent, your self-image improves, positively affecting your brain and allowing you to reclaim your mental "vibe."
- **Reduces your blood sugar:** High concentrations of sugar in the bloodstream significantly hinder the growth of the hippocampus, insular cortex, and hypothalamus, which are all located in the brain (Edwards, 2016).
- A healthy hippocampus is associated with enhanced memory, learning, and alertness.
- **Lowers your blood pressure:** Higher pressures in your arteries interfere with blood flow to the brain, depriving it of the nutrients it needs. By reducing blood sugar levels and body fat, two risk factors for developing high blood pressure, intermittent fasting can improve vascular flow to the brain.
- **Slows neurodegeneration:** When looking at conditions such as Parkinson's and Alzheimer's, there's emerging evidence that intermittent fasting can be protective. A healthy gut is the backbone of a healthy neurologic system, and fasting enhances gut health.

The research about intermittent fasting's impact on brain function is still in its infancy. There's little to no proof at this time that fasting can improve memory in women over

50. Nevertheless, the fact that it can slow the neurodegenerative process down is a great starting point.

- **Activates the onset of autophagy:** Fasting triggers a normal cellular function called autophagy, during which your cells discard dysfunctional, damaged, internal components to regenerate new, healthier material.

Newer brain cells improve your cognition by reigniting the functions of the hypothalamus and hippocampus. The process of autophagy keeps your mind fresh and alert.

Most research showing the benefits of intermittent fasting on this self-cleaning process are animal studies, and the fasting time to produce the greatest effects was 24 hours or more, as with an alternate-day fast.

However, fasting beyond one or two days can backfire and cause more harm than good. The takeaway is this:

1. Stick to a safe fasting window of 12 to 18 hours, or up to 24 hours at the most, for now.
2. Give more time for scientific evidence to catch up with chat-room anecdotes or talk to your healthcare provider before attempting to fast for more than 24 hours.
3. Intermittent fasting is good for the brain.

Mental Clarity and Focus During Fasting

Brain fog seems to come naturally to us as we grow older, doesn't it? Symptoms of this psychological condition include disorderly thoughts that cloud the mind, increase forgetfulness, and impair mental clarity.

All versions of intermittent fasting improve mental clarity in one way or another. The fasting window leads to reduced sugar levels and enhances protection of brain structures and function.

Eating intermittently also encourages a peaceful mind, a calmer approach to stressful situations, and better mood regulation. All these factors reduce brain fog and improve mental clarity.

FASTING VERSUS NEURODEGENERATIVE DISEASES

We become increasingly vulnerable to neurodegenerative and destructive diseases as we advance in age. The resulting disorders and their conventional treatment can tax the body and mind.

According to Phillips (2019), intermittent fasting can offer protection from this predicament. The earlier we start, the better the outcomes. Let's see how this benefit relates to a few specific conditions:

- **Brain cancer:** Restricting your intake of calories has anti-carcinogenic effects; it reduces the development of cancer cells in the body. In 2021, the International Food Information Council Foundation reported that managing weight with intermittent fasting can help to prevent cancer.

  For people who are already battling cancer, fasting has been shown to improve the body's response to the adverse effects of chemotherapy on affected brain tissue during and after treatment. It's promising to see fasting take such a prominent role in the fight against cancer.

- **Multiple sclerosis (MS):** When the body attacks itself, autoimmune changes occur that can cause various diseases. MS is one of the many conditions that can result from this neurodegenerative process. Intermittent fasting reduces the autoimmune inflammatory changes that cause MS (Gudden et al., 2021).

Currently, most of the findings supporting this claim are based on animal testing. However, experimental evidence in humans is catching up. Some recent studies suggest that the same positive effects may be achieved in people who fast.

- **Diseases related to metabolic syndrome**: Intermittent fasting can help to reduce the chances of developing obesity, diabetes, high cholesterol, and hypertension, which are risk factors for metabolic syndrome. This condition can trigger the onset of degenerative diseases such as Parkinson's, Alzheimer's, and others.
- **Stroke**: Hypertension and diabetes are two very significant risk factors for stroke. Excess circulating glucose can inflame blood vessels and cause pressure to rise. Intermittent fasting regulates sugar, thus reducing pressure and stroke risk.

Fasting also enhances neuroprotection and helps the body reduce oxidative stress in the brain. These two benefits contribute to a reduction in stroke risk.

- **Epilepsy**: Regular fasting helps to balance and normalize the brain's electrical activity, thus preventing the loss of conscious movement that can result in seizures. These involuntary spells are less likely to develop in people who fast consistently than those who don't.

NUTRIENTS FOR COGNITIVE HEALTH

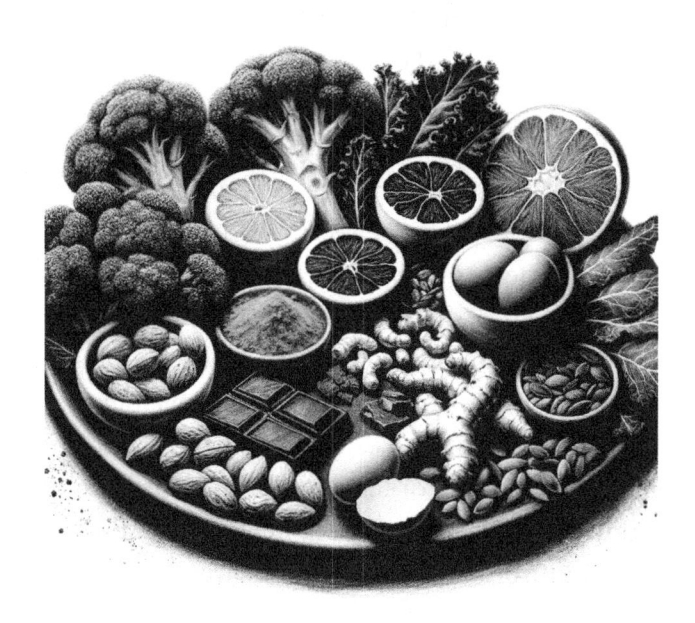

One of the keys to cognitively benefiting from intermittent fasting is to have good, basic knowledge about foods to include in your eating plan. This next section looks at the most essential nutrients in detail:

- **Carbohydrates**: This macronutrient is the body's primary fuel source; the brain utilizes a whopping 20% of it! Berries and other fruits, vegetables, and whole grains can provide the necessary carbohydrates without exceeding your daily caloric limits.
- **Micronutrients:** Vitamins and minerals are essential to brain function and integrity. Still, getting them from the diet is sometimes a struggle. Store-bought supplements that have little to no fillers or added sugar are perfect for

anyone who is fasting. To benefit fully, choose a multivitamin that has minimal calories, if any.

Also, remember to include plenty of vitamins B, D, K, E, and A in your meals. These vitamins help to keep your cognitive faculties at their best.

- **Protein:** The pathways that nerves in the brain use to communicate with each other require protein to function optimally. Include a variety of protein sources in your daily intake to meet your macros (See Chapter 2 for more information about macros). Fatty fish and lean protein are a great source; animal-free options such as tofu, complex grains, and nuts can also meet your needs.

Food and Supplements That Enhance Memory and Brain Function

The recommendations that follow are not a one-size-fits-all solution. What is helpful and practical for one person may be entirely out of the question for someone else. According to Jennings (2021) consider

- **Broccoli**: Studies conducted in older adults have linked broccoli with high cognitive ability and better memory because of its significant vitamin K content.
- **Fish:** Tuna, trout, sardines, herring, and salmon contain omega-3 fatty acids. These nutrients help to develop brain and nerve cells. Fun fact: Fat constitutes about 60% of your brain tissue, with omega-3 fatty acids making up about half of that composition.

Fish also enhances the growth of the brain's gray matter, which contains many nerve cells and regulates emotions, decision-making ability, and memory. What's good for the brain is good for the body.

- **Coffee:** This beverage contains antioxidants and caffeine that stimulate the brain and hinder the release of adenosine, which is the neurotransmitter that makes you feel drowsy. Drinking coffee during intermittent fasting improves your concentration and attention to detail.

Coffee also improves your mood by slowing elimination of the *feel-good* hormone dopamine. However, the coffee needs to be black and without any sweetener if you want to stay in a fasting state.

- **Green Tea:** For protection against cognitive decline, consider ditching the coffee and turning to green tea. In a study by Noguchi-Shinohara et al. (2014), green tea consumption outperformed coffee and black tea when it came to slowing or preventing cognitive impairment. Drink green tea without adding sweetener, cream, or milk to avoid breaking your fast.
- **Pumpkin seeds:** These oil-rich seeds contain iron, magnesium, zinc, and copper, essential in preventing neurological conditions like depression, migraines, epilepsy, Parkinson's, and Alzheimer's. Pumpkin seeds also help to prevent free radical damage to the brain's tissue.
- **Dark chocolate:** Healthier than its milky counterpart, chocolate with a higher percentage of cacao contains caffeine, flavonoids, and antioxidants, which are powerful brain boosters. Flavonoids help with memory and reduce mental decline as you grow older.
- **Turmeric:** This spice contains curcumin, the active ingredient that exerts antioxidant and anti-inflammatory

properties on the brain. Curcumin clears amyloid plaques, which are misshaped proteins that form between nerve cell spaces. This action helps to prevent memory loss associated with Alzheimer's disease.

Turmeric also helps to alleviate depression by triggering the release of dopamine and serotonin, which are mood boosters.

- **Nuts:** A diet that regularly includes nuts reduces cognitive decline as you age. Nuts contain antioxidants, vitamin E, and healthy fats for healthy brain development.
- **Eggs:** This versatile food is an excellent protein source, containing vitamins B6 and B12, choline, and folate. These nutrients are primarily concentrated in the egg yolk and are helpful in memory retention and mood regulation.

Vitamin B12 and folate deficiency can lead to depression; eggs can help.

- **Oranges:** These delectable citrus fruits contain vitamin C, which prevents mental decline and depressive brain disorders such as anxiety, Alzheimer's disease, and schizophrenia. An adequate vitamin C intake can help improve cognitive tasks like decision-making and attentive focus.

Low Glycemic Index, Anti-Inflammatory, Nutrient Dense Food Intake

To support brain health, eat meals that add nutrients to your body and improve your metabolic functions without excessive sugar or carbohydrate content. Recall that carbohydrates break down into simple sugar molecules once consumed.

How quickly your blood sugar levels shoot up after eating reflects the glycemic index or load of the food. Generally speaking, the higher the sugar content of a food, the higher its glycemic index (GI) (Harvard Health, 2019).

Conversely, low-GI foods during intermittent fasting

- **Maintain steady blood sugar for people with diabetes:** Proper planning when fasting ensures your blood glucose goes neither too high nor too low. When done correctly, intermittent fasting keeps your brain glucose and function stable during your fasting window.

Watch out for low blood sugar (hypoglycemia); it's more dangerous than hyperglycemia since it can put you in a coma. If you have diabetes, closely monitor your fasting sugars, and keep a source of glucose on hand in case of emergencies.

- **Sustain brain function:** Whole grains have components that nourish the brain and allow for stable brain-glucose levels. Steer clear of white bread, pasta, rice, or potatoes as they spike and drop sugar levels quickly. In addition, they offer less nutrition than whole grains.
- **Lower your risk of developing dementia**: Foods with a low GI decrease your likelihood of developing dementia by improving your insulin sensitivity. Enhanced insulin sensitivity helps reduce the chances of rapid brain shrinkage. Preserved brain size helps to maintain your cognition as you age (Edwards, 2016).

Just because a food has a low GI doesn't necessarily make it a good choice for your diet. Iceberg lettuce has the same GI but is less nutrient-dense than broccoli.

Some foods may have a high GI and still be nutritious at the same time. Pure, fresh-squeezed orange juice contains many essential nutrients. However, as little as four ounces still has a relatively high GI.

Focus your diet on unprocessed or whole foods while limiting the intake of simple carbohydrates, fast foods, and high-GI fruits. Doing so will improve your body's cognitive response to intermittent fasting.

Determine the macronutrients each food can deliver per serving and then plan your meals accordingly. And do not neglect dietary fat! It plays a vital role in maintaining the brain's neuronal membrane structure.

Starting an intermittent fasting routine may seem scary if you've never done it before. However, with the beneficial returns of intermittent fasting that I've shared in this chapter, you don't need to worry. Apply the nuggets we discussed and be patient with yourself. Slow and steady wins the race!

A healthy mind and a fit body are synonymous with a healthy heart when you're over 50. Cardiac benefits are explored and explained in the next chapter. Continue to dig in!

STRENGTHEN YOUR HEART

My family's health history includes cardiovascular disease, diabetes, and stroke. As you can imagine, I certainly don't want any of those things! Over the years, I've used intermittent fasting to rewrite my health story by restoring my blood sugar and cholesterol to safe levels.

Taxing as this has been, it was worth it! I hope my journey will inspire you to implement the changes needed to experience a new lease on life.

My heart disease risk is lower than average now, and seeing those improvements has been so exciting. I'm proudly modeling what it means to adopt a healthy lifestyle for my family.

Having the tools I need to take better care of myself as I age is gratifying. My lifestyle has become part of a solution, not a problem. If can do it, you can do it!

UNDERSTANDING HEART HEALTH IN WOMEN OVER 50

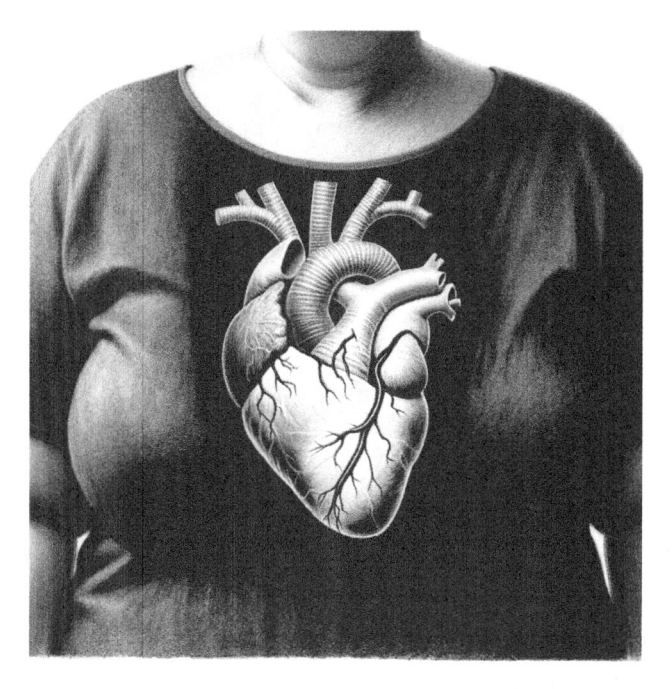

Heart disease is one of the top causes of death, particularly among women. This statement may sound a bit extreme, but it gives you something to think about as a woman in or past her 50s.

Some of the most common conditions affecting post-menopausal women include

- **Coronary artery disease:** This vascular disorder is the most common heart condition in women. It occurs when the arteries become clogged with plaque or blood clots, causing blood pressure to increase and impede blood flow. Over time, the heart muscle struggles to get the blood it needs to function normally. When this happens, a heart attack or death can follow.

- **Arrhythmia:** A heart that beats either too fast or too slow is said to be arrhythmic; this is taxing to the heart and increases the risk of forming blood clots.
- **Heart failure:** When a heart weakens, it struggles to pump blood to the body's organs, and the fluid in the circulatory system becomes too much for the heart to handle. Such a scenario may lead to organs collapsing or even to death.

Often, symptoms of a cardiac disorder are vague in women and very easy to dismiss; they don't always present like a crushing pain in the chest.

Instead, you may notice general symptoms such as difficulty breathing, sweating profusely, and constantly feeling exhausted or drained. You may have neck pain that rides along the jaw and shoulder, upper back pain, heartburn, vomiting, and indigestion.

If you've had one or more of the symptoms described in the previous paragraph, get a check-up as soon as possible to ensure no underlying problems like heart disease. Talk to your healthcare provider about *any* symptoms you experience; don't blow them off!

Unfortunately, many of you have encountered inattentive healthcare providers who don't take your symptoms seriously. Be persistent in your quest to get appropriate evaluation and treatment. Whatever you do, don't tell yourself that it's all in your head! Your intuition is a God-given tool in your armament to help keep you safe.

Common Risk Factors

It's necessary to understand heart disease risk factors so that you know what to look out for. Though this will seem like a bit of doom and gloom, there's hope for turning things around. Let's get down to it.

- **Age:** The risk of cardiovascular disease increases with aging because the vessels in your heart and body gradually weaken over time. As a healthcare provider, I strongly encourage routine checkups (not just sick visits), a healthy diet, and daily physical activity to mitigate this risk. These preventive measures are beneficial for all patients.

Rosario's 2021 blog provides some perspective by pointing out that 45% of women over 50 are at risk of heart disease. In contrast, only 10% are at risk for breast cancer.

Considering that each of us probably knows at least one woman who has battled breast cancer, this is a sobering statistic! It highlights the fact that more than four out of every ten women we know are on their way to a significant cardiac event if they don't turn things around.

Instead of being frightened by these numbers, let's take action and lead by example!

- **Stress and depression:** It's harder to maintain a healthy lifestyle and take care of yourself when feeling worn down and unmotivated. Frequent high stress and anxiety levels can lead to heart disease as they cause the body to release cortisol.

This hormone increases the cardiac workload, which requires increased blood flow (American Heart Association, 2021). An unhealthy heart won't have the stamina to keep pace. Over time, this mismatch of supply and demand is detrimental to your health.

- **Menopause:** As estrogen levels go down, so does the cardiac protection that it offers. When coupled with the finding that blood vessels become stiffer and narrower with age, the risk for heart disease increases.
- **Smoking:** Nicotine causes blood vessels to constrict, reduces circulating oxygen in the blood to the tissues, and interferes with normal blood-gas exchange in the lungs.
- **A sedentary lifestyle:** Sustained inactivity leads to sluggish circulation. Further, excessive or prolonged sitting can cause the veins in your legs to become inefficient at pumping blood back up to the heart. These changes increase your risk of blood clots, heart attack, and stroke.
- **Genetics:** A family history of heart disease at an early age puts you at risk. Other hereditary risk factors include close family members with hypertension, high cholesterol, and other cardiovascular disorders.
- **Inflammatory diseases:** Conditions such as arthritis threaten women's heart health. According to Rath (2022), your body releases inflammatory substances when you have arthritis and other chronic diseases that destroy blood vessels. These substances worsen the buildup of plaque; in turn, blood vessels narrow— eventually leading to high blood pressure and heart disease.

The Impact of Intermittent Fasting on Cardiovascular Health

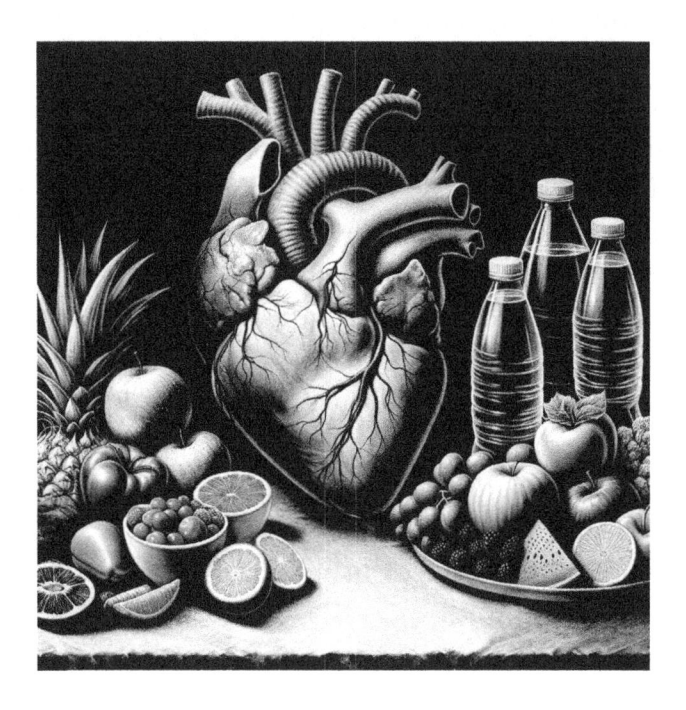

Perhaps you're questioning the link between heart health and intermittent fasting. The following information will open your mind to how a fasting regimen can enhance cardiac function.

Intermittent fasting creates suitable conditions for a ketogenic state—which lowers cardiovascular risks. Following the depletion of carbohydrate stores during a fast, your body goes into ketosis, a process that burns fat. If you are like me, you've got fat to burn!

The good news doesn't just stop there! Recall that intermittent fasting also reduces circulating blood sugar and enhances cognition. A natural result of these improvements is less inflammation and stress on the cardiovascular system and reduced overall stress on the body.

Safety Considerations for Women With Heart Conditions

While studies do show benefits of intermittent fasting on heart health, practice caution to avoid complications. One safety measure is to keep your routine fasting under 24 hours.

For added protection, make sure that you stay thoroughly hydrated. Also, avoid overexertion during a fast, which may strain and damage your heart.

Schedule a consultation with your healthcare provider before fasting to uncover any comorbidities that could increase your chances of a poor outcome. Be attentive to your body and note any new symptoms, no matter how small. Also, seek medical help if you feel ill during your fasting window.

HEART-HEALTHY NUTRITION AND FASTING

Given the seriousness of postmenopausal risk for heart disease, it's wise to keep your fast as clean as possible by eliminating all sugary and processed foods. Think of it like this: Everything you eat and drink either promotes or hinders your wellbeing.

The key to making nutritious choices that benefit your cardiovascular health is to incorporate a wide variety of healthy food into each meal. There's a popular diet that does this very well; let's take a look.

The Pesco-Mediterranean Diet

This heart-healthy fare combines multi-grains, fruits, seeds, vegetables, olive oil, spices, and legumes with seafood; making it an ideal eating plan for optimal heart health. When combined with intermittent fasting, the Mediterranean diet packs a powerful punch.

Note that the traditional Mediterranean diet limits the intake of poultry, eggs, and dairy. Absent are sugar, processed meats, refined grains, red meat, spirit alcohols, beer, and cocktails.

While the food is fantastic for your health, a beautiful takeaway from the culture is the practice of sharing. Mediterranean people share their food and eat together, enjoying nothing but each other's company without the distractions of screens and devices.

A relaxed eating environment benefits your health, especially the mental aspect.

Low glycemic index (GI) foods are typical in the Mediterranean diet, and a priority for women with underlying heart problems. Food combinations and recipes are widely available in cookbooks and online.

Low Glycemic Index Foods and Your Heart

Recall that GI relates to how quickly a food or drink raises blood sugar after consumption. The lower a food's GI, the less likely it is to contribute to changes that can lead to increased blood pressure and cardiac risk. According to Coyle (2017) the factors used to determine the rating of a food's GI include

- **Types of sugar:** Common sugars found in foods include fructose, sucrose, dextrose, and maltose. Fructose has an index of about 23, which is low compared 105 for maltose.
- **The structure of the starch:** Simple carbohydrates contain a higher percentage of amylopectin, which has a structure that is very easily digestible. The easier the digestion, the

higher the GI and the faster the starch is absorbed into the bloodstream.

However, complex carbohydrates contain more amylose. This starch is harder to digest and is slowly absorbed into the bloodstream.

Many foods that naturally have complex starches are ruined by manufacturing processes that disrupt the structure of their starch. This causes them to absorb too quickly to impart much nutritional benefit.

- **The composition of nutrients:** A food's composition determines the rate at which digestion and absorption occur. Junk food like baked goods and chips are notorious for being more 'fluff' than substance; albeit, tasty fluff.

All joking aside, these foods speed through the digestive system, pushing sugar levels high but offering little else.

- **The cooking time:** Overcooking food increases its index score because the heat makes sugars more easily digestible and rapidly absorbed into the bloodstream.
- **Ripeness of a fruit:** Have you noticed that the riper a fruit gets, the sweeter it becomes? Not only does sweetness increase, but the GI does, too. Coyle's 2017 article notes that an unripe banana scores 30 on the scale while an overripe banana is ranked 18 points higher, at 48.

Tips for Incorporating Heart-Protective Nutrients Into Meals

Try not to feel overwhelmed when incorporating heart-protective foods into your diet. As mentioned earlier, the Mediterranean diet is well-researched and endorsed as a heart-healthy option.

There is no need to abandon your cultural and customary foods, either. Include traditional items in meal planning that have a low GI, and adjust portion sizes to stay within your macros.

My parents are from the Caribbean, and plantains are an Island delicacy. I like to eat them very ripe, but the glycemic index is so high that I have to limit myself to about one-third of a cup. Though fried plantains are delicious, piercing the skin and placing them whole in an air-fryer cuts down on fat while maintaining the taste I crave.

Find ways to enjoy the foods you love without increasing cardiac risk. As a clinician, I routinely advise patients to eliminate sugary drinks and soda, limit juice servings to no more than four ounces per day, and reduce portion sizes of carbohydrates to the amount they would serve a 5-year-old child.

This strategy creates a visual representation that resonates with many people. The final portion amounts to about one-quarter of the serving size most of us would put on our dinner plates.

As mentioned previously, limit simple carbohydrates to no more than half a cup or four ounces per three to four hours. That time-frame gives the body a chance to process the sugar content of your meal without being overwhelmed.

Sugar that remains in the bloodstream can damage tissue wherever the blood flows. Nerve damage leads to neuropathy and retinopathy; kidney damage leads down the path toward dialysis, and so on.

Armed with all of this information, I am confident you would succeed if you were to start your intermittent fasting journey today. However, be ready to develop patience and dedication to achieving the desired results. Pace yourself!

Also, consult with a medical practitioner before starting a fasting program to avoid exacerbating health problems you might have, even if you don't have symptoms. When done correctly, fasting can become a healthy, life-long habit; continue to the next chapter to learn how.

LONG-TERM BENEFITS EQUALS SUCCESS

I was desperate seven years ago when I started my intermittent fasting journey. Severe overload anxiety, working full-time, and juggling clinical rotations was causing severe gastric distress. The best available treatment at the time was a costly medication that I couldn't afford.

I tried supplements, vitamins, and elimination diets with little to no success. My last-ditch effort was intermittent fasting, and it worked.

Over the past year, I've optimized my nutritional intake with intermittent fasting, lost over 20 pounds, and kept them off with a sustainable effort. Now, I'm excited to see what else is possible!

My story shows that both short-term and long-term improvements come with intermittent fasting. If you manage to keep up with your fasting routine, chances are high that you'll have the same results.

With fasting, you'll develop a resilient mind and reduce your risks for some of the conditions that are common as we get older, including cardiovascular disease, dementia, depression, stress, and anxiety. This chapter will shed more light on these and other extended benefits.

INTERMITTENT FASTING, HEALTHY AGING, AND LONGEVITY

Mental and physical improvements result from a consistent fasting regimen. These two areas of health are intertwined; the mental benefits you experience will positively affect your physical body and vice versa. We've discussed many of these gains in previous chapters - here, we will bring them together.

Your physiologic abilities will naturally decline as you age because some organs will no longer function at their best. However, intermittent fasting can help to slow down or reduce the negative impacts of some of these changes.

With structured fasting, you can develop resilience while promoting longevity. Let's explore this idea in greater detail. Intermittent fasting

- **Promotes Cell Regeneration and Tissue Growth:** By reducing oxidative stress in your tissues, fasting promotes cellular repair. It also facilitates the preservation of your skeletal muscle mass. Those muscles offer protection from falls and help you to carry out critical physical tasks.
- **Increases Release of Essential Hormones:** Human growth hormone (HGH) is responsible for repairing and promoting the growth of muscle tissues. Its release naturally declines as you get older. However, fasting increases HGH, thereby revitalizing your physical body and strength.

- **Reduces Body Fat:** As you grow older, excess body fat increases your chances of developing several conditions, including hypertension, cancer, diabetes, and heart disease. You can shed extra pounds and reduce your risk of these diseases with a fasting regimen.
- **Lowers Chances of Developing Insulin Resistance:** By increasing insulin sensitivity in your body, fasting combats resistance and helps to control the glucose levels in your blood.
- **Provides Digestive System Rest:** By giving the gut the time it needs to rest and rejuvenate, fasting reduces the risk of developing stomach issues such as diarrhea, bloating, and gas buildup. These digestive problems can cause physical discomfort, leading to anxiety and depression if they become chronic.
- **Improves Sensitivity:** As you age, the sensitivity of your tastebuds decreases. Intermittent fasting can make the buds more sensitive, which will enhance the eating experience and allow you to enjoy healthier, low sodium food.

The Psychological and Emotional Advantages of Fasting

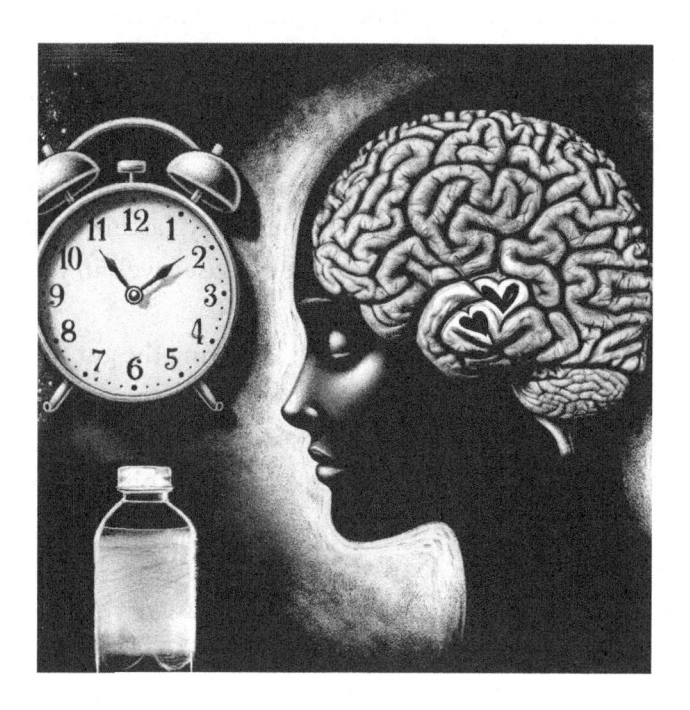

Intermittent fasting positively influences your mental state. If you adopt it as a lifestyle, some of the psychological and emotional benefits you'll enjoy are:

- **Fulfillment and contentment through improved social connections:** Fasting clears your mind and helps to reduce stressful emotions like worry and anxiety. Aging is often synonymous with social isolation and loneliness, which can lead to feelings of despair.

  A fasting regimen reduces chronic brain inflammation and mental morbidity by increasing neuron activity. These changes make it easier for you to initiate and maintain social connections.

- **Greater relaxation:** Cognitive decline and conditions like Alzheimer's disease cause disrupted sleep patterns and the inability to rest. Intermittent fasting helps you relax, improving sleep and rest.
- **Improved self-control and discipline:** With intermittent fasting, you gradually develop the ability to control your urges. This self-discipline allows you to eat what supports your health and avoid what subtracts from it, improving your overall well-being.
- **Activated systems for longevity:** Intermittent fasting reduces leptin resistance, which allows the body to burn more fat. This fat-burning improves your cognitive functions and ability to concentrate, thereby contributing to longevity.

Tips for Maintaining Motivation and Commitment to Fasting

Intermittent fasting can be a struggle for beginners. Still, it isn't impossible if you put your mind to it. Hopefully, the following tips will help you to remain enthusiastic and committed to fasting.

Set Realistic Targets: The idea of achieving your targeted body weight and shape is motivating. However, you'll need more than a weight loss goal to keep you engaged. Routines quickly become boring for anyone, and some results of intermittent fasting may take weeks to months to become visibly noticeable.

Realistic long-term targets will help you to stay motivated.

I initially gave myself six months to shed 20-25 pounds and keep it off for good. There were many ups and downs along the way, and I had to lengthen my projected time due to frequent travels. Nevertheless, it was a still a realistic goal, and I made it!

Create an Exciting Reward System: To prevent boredom, incorporate strategies for rewarding yourself each time you complete your fast. For example, treat yourself to a movie or favorite TV show, or a soothing bubble bath. After maintaining your intermittent fasting routine for an entire month, you could get a pedicure or manicure, take a short trip, or have a "staycation."

Just find something that makes you feel good about your achievement, and do it!

Break Goals Into Smaller Steps: Your fasting goal might be to achieve a trim and toned body or to keep a condition like anxiety or depression under control. These are generally broad goals that can be broken down into smaller steps so that you can assess and reward your progress.

For example, you can divide the total weight you want to lose into smaller amounts you aim to shed monthly or weekly. I prefer to focus on clothes fitting looser instead of watching the scale because weight fluctuates daily regardless of what you do. Those frequent changes can be confusing and discouraging if you are checking too often.

When you increase physical activity and hydration as recommended in previous chapters, the scale may initially show appropriate weight gain. If you don't consider that muscle weighs more than fat, you'll feel defeated when the numbers go up.

For the reasons just mentioned, I think it's much better to have an inspirational item of clothing like a pair of non-stretchy pants or a tight bra that you try to squeeze into once weekly. As your body starts trimming down, that clothing will become looser, so keep it up! Soon, you'll have a good reason to go on a shopping spree!

If mood stabilization is your goal, why not write down what achieving this goal would look like and itemize the steps? For some people, a goal of joining a local organization might start with researching what's available or asking around at work or church.

Each endeavor requires a step-wise approach; achieving those steps is worth celebrating. Whatever you do, make it easy to recognize and reward success. These smaller, measurable objectives will help to prevent burnout.

Monitor Progress by How You Feel: The mental benefits of fasting tend to appear well before the physical benefits. Set yourself up for mini-victories along the journey.

I use an app that gives a celebratory animation whenever I stay within my allotted carbohydrate, fat, and protein macros, and calories. The app provides four daily opportunities for me to succeed and feel good. The achievements keep me excited and motivated.

Avoid Comparing Yourself to Others: Comparing yourself with the next person can demotivate you if it seems they're getting better results. Instead, focus on your progress by being aware of your body's unique needs and striving to meet them. Look for improvements in your lab values, energy levels, and mental clarity to understand better how fasting works for you.

Incorporate Exercises to Promote Success: Even a mild increase in physical activity enhances the effects of fasting so you can experience the results much quicker. Exercise improves your overall well-being, which should boost your enthusiasm.

CREATING A SUSTAINABLE FASTING ROUTINE

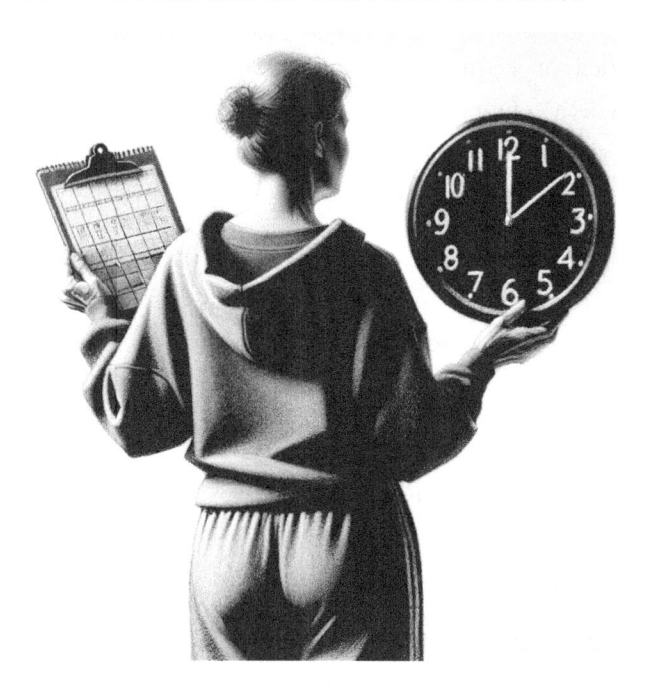

When you reach the age of 50, hormonal shifts will likely cause changes to your physical abilities and limits. Your nutrient requirements will also differ from what they were in your 40s. These two factors can make sustaining your previously managed activities and routines challenging.

Choose a fasting regimen that your schedule and body can handle. If your current fasting interval is frustrating or harming you in any way, be it psychologically or physically, change it or take a break for a while.

Here are a few more tips to help you find a sustainable plan:

- **Adjust your interval as needed:** Once you select a fasting routine to follow, remember that you can change it when needed. If 18 hours is too disruptive to your daily routine

or lifestyle, switch to the 16:8 or 14:10 version rather than quit fasting altogether.
- **Monitor your eating window:** Space your meals evenly during eating windows to maximize protein-sparing (see Chapter 3). Minimize the loss of muscle mass by consuming adequate protein, healthy fats, and complex carbohydrates at metabolically advantageous times throughout the day.
- **Track your nutrient intake:** Keep a food log for one to two weeks to review your intake before adjusting your fasting routine. Sometimes, the issue may be that your diet is leaving you malnourished. This can make it difficult to obtain enough energy to support yourself through fasting.

If you've tried using a macro calculator but failed, see your healthcare provider or a nutritionist for an evaluation. There may be an underlying issue or condition that is hindering your progress.

- **Keep the menu in check when eating out:** It's easy to lose sight of your fasting routine and get carried away at restaurants. Avoid falling into this trap by checking the menu in advance for options that support your fasting goals.

Alternatively, ask for a to-go box as soon as the food is delivered to your table. Split the meal immediately so you can have another 'take-out' meal later in the week.

Incorporate Flexibility Without Compromising Results

A flexible mindset can help you to navigate work and other commitments while staying on course with your fasting regimen.

You won't need to quit fasting if you can adapt quickly and easily. Try applying one or both of the following tips:

- **Break your fast into smaller periods:** If regular commitments keep getting in the way of your fasting routine, consider a 5:2 fast that includes one weekend day and a weekday when the demands are lowest.

  Alternatively, see if a 12:12 or 14:10 fast is more to your liking.

- **Prepare your meals in advance:** Your busy schedule can derail your fasting plans. This money and time-saving strategy is a great solution, and it works even better if you do all of your meal and snack preparation on one day.

I typically spend Sunday afternoons with a book on tape, a soup pot, a wide variety of fruits and vegetables, my juicer, blender, vacuum sealer, and chopping board. Two to three hours later I'm set for the week!

Strategies for Managing Social Events and Holidays While Fasting

Attending social events and gatherings or being away from home during your fast may be challenging. Nevertheless, advanced planning can help you stick to your routine. Try one or more of these strategies:

- **Select venues that accommodate special orders:** Restaurants may sometimes allow special, off-menu orders that match your stipulated requirements. Otherwise, fruit, salads, soups, and steamed vegetable sides can help you stay on track. Try not to go for refills on things like bread and drinks.

If all else fails, order appetizers, ask for a to-go box and split the meal, or share a meal with your travel companion(s). At social or holiday events, load up on foods from the vegetable, protein, and fruit platters before heading over to the bread, dessert, and drink tables.

- **Prepare your meals:** Whenever possible, select a vacation rental that has a kitchen so that you can prepare your meals. Set aside a morning or afternoon to visit a local deli for easy-to-prepare dishes. If that is not realistic, try controlling the things that you can.

Most hotel rooms have a mini fridge, so purchase snacks, boiled eggs, cheese, fruit, and chopped vegetables to supplement restaurant and room-order food. Travel with dry food items that help you stick to your eating plan but might not be available at your destination.

- **Communicate clearly:** Excusing yourself from a meal that everyone else is having can be challenging, and doing so may give the impression that you don't want to socialize. Explain that you are fasting or following a diet that requires you to pass on some of the food offered.

Intermittent fasting helps you achieve a healthier body and mind, with many other long-term benefits you won't want to miss. To increase your chances of enjoying the rewards, be flexible and take steps to remain motivated.

Find ways to enjoy the journey and maintain gains for life.

CONCLUSION

The various forms of intermittent fasting differ based on the lengths of the eating and fasting windows. This flexibility makes it easy for you to choose the best method based on your schedule, type of work, and workout routines, among other factors.

A long-term fasting regimen can offset some of the negative changes associated with aging. It gives the digestive system time to absorb nutrients, rest, and rejuvenate. Gut health is linked to brain, heart, and organ health. The positive impact of intermittent fasting on various body functions cannot be overstated.

Starting with Chapter 1, we've seen intermittent fasting as an effective weight loss tool, especially when combined with proper nutrition and exercise. I've offered many strategies to help you start and succeed with a fasting plan while navigating plateaus and stalls.

In short, I've removed all your objections to beginning your intermittent fasting journey. You are your best cheerleader: Tell yourself that you can do it!

Even after reading this book, continue to make efforts that lead to self-discovery and greater confidence with intermittent fasting. I wish you a healthier and happier life!

∼

MAKE A DIFFERENCE WITH YOUR REVIEW
UNLOCK THE POWER OF INTERMITTENT FASTING

Please take a moment to scan the QR below to share your thoughts so others can find my book :-)

FREQUENTLY ASKED QUESTIONS

1. How should I approach fasting as a diabetic on insulin? Before starting an intermittent fasting regimen, go for a clinical visit and lab testing. Work with your healthcare provider to determine your goal sugar level, and talk about how to recognize if your sugar is running low and what to do about it.

Low blood sugar is dangerous and can lead to a coma or death. Intermittent fasting may still be an option, but you will need to be supervised by your healthcare provider.

2. What breaks the fast? Any caloric intake breaks a fast. That doesn't necessarily mean that you lose all the benefits you gained. Benefits are maintained to some degree, assuming you stick to your intermittent fasting schedule most of the time, follow a healthy diet, and adequately manage stress.

3. What is clean fasting versus dirty fasting? A clean fast is a calorie-free fast in which you consume only water. A dirty fast incorporates foods or drinks that will kick you out of the fasting state but don't add significant calories.

As little as a tablespoon of milk or cream, a teaspoon of olive oil, or an ounce of protein provides an external fuel source. Your body will burn them for energy instead of fat.

Even if you don't consume anything else for hours, you won't re-enter a fat-burning state until at least 12 hours of no caloric intake.

4. What about taking medication and supplements when fasting? Many medications do not add calories and will not break a fast. However, medicated syrups have calories. Many supplements are packed with fillers that can add calories.

Some supplement manufacturers list the calorie count on the back of the bottle or packaging so you can see it, but not all. When in doubt, wait until you break your fast to take supplements, but take all medications as prescribed.

5. Does adding lemon juice or lime to water break a fast? Anything that has calories can break a fast. Some sources say if you stay under ten calories, you're not breaking a fast; others say even one calorie breaks a fast. If you want to be sure, I recommend drinking only water or herbal tea without sweeteners. Alternatively, try a tablespoon of apple cider vinegar or one to two drops of food-grade citrus essential oil in a full glass of water.

6. What conditions can intermittent fasting make worse? If not done correctly, fasting can aggravate diabetes. Low sugar, also known as hypoglycemia, is a concerning possibility for people with diabetes. Before starting with intermittent fasting, know your A1c and fasting sugar levels.

If you haven't been able to consistently keep your fasting sugars in the goal range, don't start intermittent fasting without first consulting with your healthcare provider.

Fasting can aggravate other conditions, including insomnia. Check out Chapter 1 for more information about who should and should not do intermittent fasting.

7. My breath stinks; what can I do? Try a swish and spit mouthwash or use film breath fresheners. Try adding a drop of food-grade peppermint, citrus, or lavender oil to a glass of water. Maintain adequate hydration, and consider drinking apple cider vinegar water (one tablespoon to a full glass of water).

8. What if I don't like vegetables? Soups are a great place to hide vegetables. Check out the soup recipe in Chapter 4. Many healthy shake recipes call for fruits and vegetables for a smooth and tasty treat.

9. Will fasting make hot flashes go away? Research findings are divided: some say intermittent fasting can help, while others say it can trigger hot flashes. Nevertheless, the myriad of health benefits associated with intermittent fasting makes it a worthwhile endeavor for menopausal women, even if it doesn't impact hot flashes.

10. How should I break a fast? During your fasting hours, your body has been using fat for fuel. If you want to keep that process going, break your fast with water or tea and a source of protein; hold off on fatty foods and carbs for a while longer. Of course, if you're going to work or working out, add healthy carbs to fuel your increased activity.

11. How should I handle cravings? Postpone eating or giving in as long as possible to stick to your fasting interval. Drink water with or without apple cider vinegar; drink an herbal tea or black coffee. Chapters 2, 3, and 4 have a lot of strategies and tips that can help.

12. I've been fasting for five weeks and haven't lost weight; what am I doing wrong? First, rule out health conditions with a visit to your healthcare provider. Second, look at how your clothes are fitting - especially the band of your bra and the waist of your pants. A looser fit means you are on the right track.

Daily exercise can speed up the weight loss process, though muscle weighs more than fat and may cause your weight to increase initially. Recall that intermittent fasting also conveys various health benefits that lead to longevity, better brain and heart health, etc.

It's not just about the weight loss in terms of the benefits you gain.

13. How will I know how much to eat? Use an intermittent fasting or macros app that helps you track your food intake. The CarbManager app is my favorite because it is very user-friendly. I used it to enter my starting and ideal weights, and it calculated the calorie deficit I would need to achieve my goal. The app allowed me to customize my percentages of carbohydrates, fat, and protein using information obtained from a free online macro calculator.

Check out Chapter 2 for more details on macro percentages.

14. How can I incorporate fasting if I am a shift worker? Try scheduling your day as if you were not a shift worker. If you go straight to bed upon returning home, have your last meal at work three hours before quitting time. Chapter 3 discusses strategies for shift workers; check it out.

15. How do I figure out my eating window? Try to break your fast during the first one to two hours of work, school, or other physically demanding activities. For example, if you work 5 a.m. to 1 p.m. for a typical eight-hour day, you might break your fast at 6 a.m.; eight hours later, at 2 p.m., you would start fasting again for a 16:8 regimen.

A more straightforward method is to start counting fasting hours after your last meal the day prior. Let's say you go out to dinner with friends, and the last piece of food passes your lips at 8 p.m. If you plan to do a 14 to 16-hour fast, your first meal the next day should take place between 10 a.m. and noon.

16. Should I keep the same fasting interval all the time, or change it? Research shows the best results when you change up your fasting intervals. Think of it as tricking your body so it doesn't get used to one thing. We want our bodies to adapt.

17. Will intermittent fasting increase my sugar levels? It shouldn't. A known or unknown health condition could be the problem. A diet with inadequate protein or fiber could be contributory. Both protein and fiber help to keep blood sugar levels steady. Talk to your healthcare provider before proceeding further with fasting, as a precaution.

18. How can I get back on track after taking a trip? You can compensate for some lost time by doing a more intensive intermittent fast for a week (18:6 plus clean eating, for example). Some people prefer to drop to one meal a day for a short time or do an alternate-day fast for one to two weeks before returning to their usual fasting regimen.

Increasing exercise intensity while maintaining your usual fasting schedule is another way to get back on track.

19. What about OMAD for intermittent fasting? By eating only one meal a day, you'll take in only one-third to one-half of your usual calories within one hour, then you will fast the rest of the time, anywhere from 22-23 hours. Research shows that people tend to gain weight back after about six months of OMAD alone, likely because it's too demanding to sustain.

Try it for one to two weeks, then switch to an 18:6 or 16:8 fast for a few weeks. Go back to OMAD once a month to see if doing so provides lasting results.

20. I am not making any progress; what can I do? Weight loss is a slow and long process because we are trying to change decades of behavior and cell memory. Slow and steady wins the race. A lot of the battle takes place in the mind. Approach plateaus on your fasting journey with introspection, focusing on six areas:

> **A. What you think about yourself:** Address self-doubt, poor self-esteem, and lack of confidence through journaling, prayer, and affirmations. I use mostly Bible verses that inspire and encourage; they help me through tough times and plateaus.
> **B. What you think about food:** Journal what you eat and drink, your mood when you eat, and afterward. Over time, you'll see the connections worth strengthening and those that need breaking. You may need counseling for these two steps. Give yourself permission and patience to get the support you need.
> **C. What you eat and drink:** You're safe following the Mediterranean diet as it's well-researched and has many resources online.
> **D. Sleep quality and stress:** Keep stress levels as low as possible; eliminate or reduce noises, lights, and other distractions within an hour of sleep time.
> **E. Exercise:** Do what you can, whether it's chair exercises, walking, body weight exercises, dancing, or going to the gym; just get moving!
> **F. Non-weight benefits:** It may take 4-6 weeks for your body to start taking you seriously, but stick to it. Even

though you may not see changes on the scale, a lot is happening behind the scenes:

- The risk of heart disease is lowering.
- There is less free radical damage to cells.
- Blood sugar is going down.
- Cells are living longer.
- Fat is being burned for fuel.
- Fat cells are getting smaller.

REFERENCES

Adelson, K. I. (2022, September 30). *4 tips for building muscle and burning fat after menopause*. Tonal. https://www.tonal.com/blog/losing-weight-after menopause/

Akesson, A. (2017, July 22). *"I am feeling better than I have in years."* Diet Doctor. https://www.dietdoctor.com/feeling-better-years

Alzheimer's Disease Research Center. (2020, October 8). *Intermittent fasting and its effects on the brain*. https://www.adrc.wisc.edu/dementia-matters/intermittent-fasting-and-its-effects-brain

American Heart Association Editorial Staff. (2021, June 22). *How does depression affect the heart?* American Heart Association. https://www.heart.org/en/healthy-living/healthy-lifestyle/mental-health-and-wellbeing/how-does-depression-affect-the-heart

Asp, K. (2023, March 2). *Fact or fiction? Assessing 8 common intermittent fasting myths*. Woman's World. https://www.womansworld.com/posts/health/eight-common-intermittent-fasting-myths

Bangkok Dusit Medical Services. (n.d.). *Brain fog: Solutions to help you improve concentration*. Bangkok Hospital. https://www.bangkokhospital.com/en/content/brain-fog-syndrome

Bassett, J. H. D., & Williams, G. R. (2016). Role of thyroid hormones in skeletal development and bone maintenance. *Endocrine Reviews, 37*(2), 135–187. https://doi.org/10.1210/er.2015-1106

Batayneh, R. (2022, September 28). *The health benefits of a whole foods diet*. Martha Stewart. https://www.marthastewart.com/7988488/health-benefits-whole-foods-based-diet

Behl, M. S. (2019, May 1). *Lab tests before you begin intermittent fasting for weight loss*. Sepalika. https://sepalika.com/intermittent-fasting/lab-tests-needed-for-a-successful-intermittent-fasting-weight-loss-program/

Bell, J. (2022, December 12). *Kale pasta sauce*. A Sweet Alternative. https://www.asweetalternative.com/blog/kale-pasta-sauce

Bell, J. (2023, September 4). *Fig cookies*. A Sweet Alternative. https://www.asweetalternative.com/blog/fig-cookies

Belman, O. (2019, April 18). *Eat less, live longer? The science of fasting and longevity*. USC Leonard Davis School of Gerontology. https://gero.usc.edu/2019/04/18/eat-less-live-longer-the-science-of-fasting-and-longevity/

REFERENCES

Bellar, D., Glickman, E. L., Judge, L. W., & Gunstad, J. (2013, June 24). Serum ghrelin is associated with verbal learning and adiposity in a sample of healthy, fit, older adults. *BioMed Research International, 2013, Article ID 202757, 5 pages.* https://dx.doi.org/10.1155/2013/202757

Benjet, C., Bromet, E., Karam, E. G., Kessler, R. C., McLaughlin, K. A., Ruscio, A. M., Shahly, V., Stein, D. J., Petukhova, M., Hill, E., Alonso, J., Atwoli, L., Bunting, B., Bruffaerts, R., Caldas-de-Almeida, J. M., de Girolamo, G., Florescu, S., Gureje, O., Huang, Y., & Lepine, J. P. (2016). The epidemiology of traumatic event exposure worldwide: Results from the World Mental Health Survey Consortium. *Psychological Medicine, 46*(2), 327–343. https://doi.org/10.1017/s0033291715001981

Benton, E. (2020, April 27). *6 reasons you've hit a weight loss plateau while doing intermittent fasting.* Women's Health. https://www.womenshealthmag.com/weight-loss/a32223696/intermittent-fasting-plateau/

Berg, Eric. "Lemon Water is Essential for Fasting." Dr. Berg Blog, 11/13/23, Lemon Water is Essential for Fasting | Healthy Keto™ Dr. Berg (drberg.com). Accessed 12 December 2023.

Berthelot, E., Etchecopar-Etchart, D., Thellier, D., Lancon, C., Boyer, L., & Fond, G. (2021). Fasting interventions for stress, anxiety, and depressive symptoms: A systematic review and meta-analysis. *Nutrients, 13*(11), 3947. https://doi.org/10.3390/nu13113947

Biostrap USA. (2022, February 25). *What is mental acuity? How diet and exercise influence memory loss.* https://Biostrap.com/Academy/Mental-Acuity/. https://biostrap.com/academy/mental-acuity/

Bitsoli, S. (2022, April 13). Relieving stress during menopause. Red Hot Mamas. https://redhotmamas.org/relieving-stress-during-menopause/

Bolster, M. B. (2023, August 14). *5 things to know about osteoporosis.* MSD Manual Consumer Version. https://www.msdmanuals.com/home/news/editorial/2023/08/11/16/52/5-things-every-patient-should-know-about-osteoporosis

Buckingham, C., & 2020. (2020, September 14). *11 people who should never try intermittent fasting.* Eat This Not That. https://www.eatthis.com/is-intermittent-fasting-safe/

Byakodi, R. (2021, November 16). *Intermittent fasting plateau: 6 tips to start losing weight.* 21 Day Hero. https://21dayhero.com/intermittent-fasting-plateau/

Calculator.net. (2015). *Macro calculator.* https://www.calculator.net/macro-calculator.html

Casale, J., & Huecker, M. R. (2020). *Fasting.* PubMed; StatPearls Publishing. https://www.ncbi.nlm.nih.gov/books/NBK534877/

CDC. (2023, February 21). *Women and heart disease.* Centers for Disease Control and Prevention. https://www.cdc.gov/heartdisease/women.htm

Cherra, S. J., & Chu, C. T. (2008). Autophagy in neuroprotection and neurodegeneration: A question of balance. *Future Neurology, 3*(3), 309–323. https://doi.org/10.2217/14796708.3.3.309

Cienfuegos, S., Corapi, S., Gabel, K., Ezpeleta, M., Kalam, F., Lin, S., Pavlou, V., & Varady, K., A. (2022). Effect of Intermittent Fasting on Reproductive Hormone Levels in Females and Males: A Review of Human Trials. *Nutrients, 14*(11), 2343. https://doi.org/10.3390/nu14112343

Cleveland Clinic. (2023, September 3). *Bioidentical hormones: Side effects, uses and more.* https://my.clevelandclinic.org/health/articles/15660-bioidentical-hormones

Cleveland Clinic. (2019, April 30). *Intermittent fasting: 4 different types explained.* Health Essentials from Cleveland Clinic. https://health.clevelandclinic.org/intermittent-fasting-4-different-types-explained/

Cleveland Clinic. (2022, March 18). *Serotonin: What is it, function and levels.* https://my.clevelandclinic.org/health/articles/22572-serotonin

Cleveland Clinic. (2022b, April 21). *Ghrelin hormone: Function and definition.* https://my.clevelandclinic.org/health/body/22804-ghrelin

Cleveland Clinic. (2022, August 23). *Autophagy: Definition, process, fasting and signs.* https://my.clevelandclinic.org/health/articles/24058-autophagy

Cleveland Clinic. (2023, March 13). *How to tell when you're full (before you feel stuffed).* Health Essentials from Cleveland Clinic. https://health.clevelandclinic.org/how-to-tell-when-you-are-full

Cleveland Clinic. (2023, May 25). *Cholecystokinin: Hormone function and definition.* https://my.clevelandclinic.org/health/body/23110-cholecystokinin

Clifton, K. K., Ma, C. X., Fontana, L., & Peterson, L. L. (2021). Intermittent fasting in the prevention and treatment of cancer. *CA: A Cancer Journal for Clinicians, 71*(6), 527–546. https://doi.org/10.3322/caac.21694

Coyle, D. (2017). *A beginner's guide to the low-glycemic diet.* Healthline. https://www.healthline.com/nutrition/low-glycemic-diet

Coyle, D. (2020, June 30). *Everything you want to know about the low glycemic diet.* Healthline. https://www.healthline.com/nutrition/low-glycemic-diet

Cushman, M., Shay, C. M., Howard, V. J., Jiménez, M. C., Lewey, J., McSweeney, J. C., Newby, L. K., Poudel, R., Reynolds, H. R., Rexrode, K. M., Sims, M., & Mosca, L. J. (2020). Ten-year differences in women's awareness related to coronary heart disease: Results of the 2019 American Heart Association National Survey: A special report from the American Heart Association. *Circulation, 143*(7). https://doi.org/10.1161/cir.0000000000000907

Czarnecka, K., Pilarz, A., Rogut, A., Maj, P., Szymanska, J., Olejnik, L., & Szymanski, P. (2021). Aspartame-True or False? Narrative review of safety analysis of general use in products. *Nutrients, 13*(6), 1957. https://doi.org/10.

3390/nu13061957

Dalkin, G. (2019, March). *Really green smoothie*. EatingWell. https://www.eatingwell.com/recipe/270514/really-green-smoothie/

Damjanovic, J. (2022, February 7). *U of T experts weigh in on whether to mix intermittent fasting and exercise*. University of Toronto News. https://www.utoronto.ca/news/u-t-experts-weigh-whether-mix-intermittent-fasting-and-exercise

Davidson, K. (2021, September 20). *The definitive guide to healthy eating in your 50s and 60s*. Healthline. https://www.healthline.com/nutrition/healthy-eating-50s-60s

Dempsey, R. (2022, September 14). *3 ways to calculate basal metabolic rate*. WikiHow. https://www.wikihow.com/Calculate-Basal-Metabolic-Rate

De Paoli, M., Zahkaria, A., Werstuck, G. H. (2021). The Role of Estrogen in Insulin Resistance: A Review of Clinical and Preclinical Data. *The American Journal of Pathology, 191*(9), 1490-1498. https://doi.org/10.1016/j.ajpath.2021.05.011 https://doi.org/10.1016/j.ajpath.2021.05.011

Dhillon, K. K., & Gupta, S. (2019, April 21). *Biochemistry, ketogenesis*. National Library of Medicine. https://www.ncbi.nlm.nih.gov/books/NBK493179/

Dong, T. A., Sandesara A, P. B., Dhindsa, D. S., Mehta, A., Arnerson, L. C., Dollar, A. L., Taub, P. R., & Sperling, L. S. (2020). Intermittent fasting: A heart-healthy dietary pattern? *The American Journal of Medicine, 133*(8). https://doi.org/10.1016/j.amjmed.2020.03.030

Edwards, S. (2016). *Sugar and the brain*. Harvard Medical School. https://hms.harvard.edu/news-events/publications-archive/brain/sugar-brain

El-Zayat, S. R., Sibaii, H., & El-Shamy, K. A. (2019, December 30). Epinephrine: An overview. *Science Direct*. https://www.sciencedirect.com/topics/earth-and-planetary-sciences/epinephrine

Elam, T., & Taku, K. (2022). Differences between posttraumatic growth and resilience: Their distinctive relationships with empathy and emotion recognition ability. *Frontiers in Psychology, 13*. https://doi.org/10.3389/fpsyg.2022.825161

Elias, A., Padinjakara, N., & Lautenschlager, N. T. (2023). Effects of intermittent fasting on cognitive health and Alzheimer's disease. *Nutrition Reviews, 81*(9), 1225-1223. https://doi.org/10.1093/nutrit/nuad021

Elias, R. (2023, January 17). *3 things*. Red Ventures. https://www.redventures.com/blog/categories/3-things

Farooq, A., Herrera, C. P., Almudahka, F., & Mansour, R. (2015). A prospective study of the physiological and neurobehavioral effects of Ramadan fasting in preteen and teenage boys. *Journal of the Academy of Nutrition and Dietetics, 115*(6), 889-897. https://doi.org/10.1016/j.jand.2015.02.012

Fetters, K. A. (2015, January 2). Intermittent fasting: Should you exercise on empty? CNN. https://edition.cnn.com/2014/12/30/health/dailyburn-exercise-empty/index.html

Gkastaris, K., Goulis, D. G., Potoupnis, M., Anastasilakis, A. D., & Kapetanos, G. (2020). Obesity, osteoporosis and bone metabolism. *Journal of Musculoskeletal & Neuronal Interactions, 20*(3), 372-381

Glycemic Index Foundation. (n.d.). *GI and heart disease.* https://www.gisymbol.com/gi-and-heart-disease/

Gonzalez, J. E., & Cooke, W. H. (2022). Influence of an acute fast on ambulatory blood pressure and autonomic cardiovascular control. *American Journal of Physiology-Regulatory, Integrative and Comparative Physiology, 322*(6), R542–R550. https://doi.org/10.1152/ajpregu.00283.2021

Good Food Team. (n.d.). *Healthy porridge bowl.* Good Food. https://www.bbcgoodfood.com/recipes/healthy-porridge-bowl

Groves, M. (2018, November 23). *Menopause diet: How what you eat affects your symptoms.* Healthline. https://www.healthline.com/nutrition/menopause-diet#foods-to-avoid

Gudden, J., Arias Vasquez, A., & Bloemendaal, M. (2021). The effects of intermittent fasting on brain and cognitive function. *Nutrients, 13*(9), 3166. https://doi.org/10.3390/nu13093166

Hadi, A., Pourmasoumi, M., Najafgholizadeh, A., Clark, C. C. T., & Esmaillzadeh, A. (2021). The effect of apple cider vinegar on lipid profiles and glycemic parameters: a systematic review and meta-analysis of randomized clinical trials. *BMC Complementary Medicine and Therapies, 21*(1), 179. https://bmccomplementmedtherapies.biomedcentral.com/articles/10.1186/s12906-021-03351-w

Hameed, S., & Wasay, M. (2020). Effects of intermittent fasting on taste modulation and perception. *Pakistan Journal of Neurological Pakistan Journal of Neurological Sciences, 15*(2), 11. https://ecommons.aku.edu/cgi/viewcontent.cgi?article=1481&context=pjns

Harper-Harrison, G., & Shanahan, M. M. (2019, May 30). *Hormone replacement therapy.* National Library of Medicine. https://www.ncbi.nlm.nih.gov/books/NBK493191/

Harvard Health Publishing. (2017, May 31). *Eat only every other day and lose weight?* Harvard Medical School. https://www.health.harvard.edu/blog/eat-only-every-other-day-and-lose-weight-2017053111791

Harvard Health Publishing. (2019). *The lowdown on glycemic index and glycemic load.* Harvard Medical School. https://www.health.harvard.edu/diseases-and-conditions/the-lowdown-on-glycemic-index-and-glycemic-load

Harvard Health Publishing. (2020, August 31). *Should you try the keto diet?* Harvard Medical School. https://www.health.harvard.edu/staying-healthy/should-you-try-the-keto-diet

Harvard T. H. Chan School of Public Health. (2022, November 18). *Healthy longevity.* https://www.hsph.harvard.edu/nutritionsource/healthy-longevity/

Henderson, Y. O., Bithi, N., Link, C., Yang, J., Schugar, R., Llarena, N., Brown, J. M., & Hine, C. (2021). Late-life intermittent fasting decreases aging-related frailty and increases renal hydrogen sulfide production in a sexually dimorphic manner. *GeroScience, 43*(4), 1527–1554. https://doi.org/10.1007/s11357-021-00330-4

Herzog, H. (2023). *How chronic stress drives the brain to crave comfort food.* Garvan Institute of Medical Research. https://www.garvan.org.au/news-events/news/how-chronic-stress-drives-the-brain-to-crave-comfort-food

Hill, A. (2019, June 14). *Can you combine intermittent fasting and coffee?* Healthline. https://www.healthline.com/nutrition/intermittent-fasting-coffee

HUR. (2018, March 1). *8 effective seated exercises for seniors in wheelchairs.* HUR USA. https://hurusa.com/8-effective-seated-exercises-for-wheelchair-bound-seniors/

The importance of female friendships during menopause. (n.a., n.d.). Kindra. https://ourkindra.com/blogs/journal/the-importance-of-female-friendships-during-menopause

Jennings, K-A. (2021, June 4). *11 best foods to boost your brain and memory.* Healthline. https://www.healthline.com/nutrition/11-brain-foods

Johns Hopkins Medicine. (2021). *Intermittent fasting: What is it, and how does it work?* https://www.hopkinsmedicine.org/health/wellness-andprevention/intermittent-fasting-what-is-it-and-how-does-it-work

Johnson, J. B., Summer, W., Cutler, R. G., Martin, B., Hyun, D.-H., Dixit, V. D., Pearson, M., Nassar, M., Tellejohan, R., Maudsley, S., Carlson, O., John, S., Laub, D. R., & Mattson, M. P. (2007). Alternate-day calorie restriction improves clinical findings and reduces markers of oxidative stress and inflammation in overweight adults with moderate asthma. *Free Radical Biology and Medicine, 42*(5), 665– 674. https://doi.org/10.1016/j.freeradbiomed.2006.12.005

Joseph, S. (2009). Growth following adversity: Positive psychological perspectives on posttraumatic stress. *Psychological Topics, 18*(2), 335–344.

Kallmyer, T. (2019, April 8). *Macro calculator.* Healthy Eater. https://healthyeater.com/flexible-dieting-calculator

Keenan, S., Cooke, M. B., Chen, W. S., Wu, S., & Belski, R. (2022). The Effects of intermittent fasting and continuous energy restriction with exercise on cardiometabolic biomarkers, dietary compliance, and perceived hunger and mood: Secondary outcomes of a randomised, controlled trial. *Nutrients, 14*(15), 3071. https://doi.org/10.3390/nu14153071

Kim, B. H., Joo, Y., Kim, M.-S., Choe, H. K., Tong, Q., & Kwon, O. (2021). Effects of intermittent fasting on the circulating levels and circadian rhythms of hormones. *Endocrinology and Metabolism, 36*(4), 745–756. https://doi.org/10.3803/enm.2021.405

Koutouroushis, C., & Sarkar, O. (2021). Role of autophagy in cardiovascular disease and aging. *Cureus, 13*(11). https://doi.org/10.7759/cureus.20042

Kubala, J. (2018, July 3). *The warrior diet: Review and beginner's guide*. Healthline. https://www.healthline.com/nutrition/warrior-diet-guide

Kubala, J. (2023, March 31). *Is fasting safe for women over 50?* Mindbodygreen. https://www.mindbodygreen.com/articles/intermittent-fasting-for-women-over50

Leiva, C. (2019, March 12). *9 tips for getting enough protein during intermittent fasting*. Insider. https://www.insider.com/getting-protein-while-fasting-2019

Leonard, J. (2020, April 16). *7 ways to do intermittent fasting: Best methods and quick tips*. Medical News Today. https://www.medicalnewstoday.com/articles/322293

Licalzi, D. (2020, October 23). *How intermittent fasting impacts longevity: A summary of the research*. Inside Tracker. https://blog.insidetracker.com/intermittent-fasting-impacts-longevitysummary-research

Lindberg, S. (2020, September 1). *How to exercise safely during intermittent fasting*. Healthline. https://www.healthline.com/health/how-to-exercise-safelyintermittent-fasting

Longo, V. D., Di Tano, M., Mattson, M. P., & Guidi, N. (2021). Intermittent and periodic fasting, longevity, and disease. *Nature Aging, 1*(1), 47–59. https://doi.org/10.1038/s43587-020-00013-3

Maiuolo, J., Gliozzi, M., Musolino, V., Carresi, C., Scarano, F., Nucera, S., Scicchitano, M., Bosco, F., Ruga, S., Zito, M., Macri, R., Bulotta, R, Muscoli, C., & Mollace, V. (2021). From metabolic syndrome to neurological diseases: Role of autophagy. *Frontiers in Cell and Developmental Biology,* (9). https://www.frontiersin.org/articles/10.3389/fcell.2021.651021

Manaye, S., Kaaviya C., Murthy, C., Bornemann, E. A., Hari Krishna K., Alabbas, M., Elashahab, M., Abid, N., & Arcia, A. P. (2023). The role of high-intensity and high-impact exercises in improving bone health in postmenopausal women: A systematic review. *Cureus*. https://doi.org/10.7759/cureus.34644

Mattson, M. P., Longo, V. D., & Harvie, M. (2017). Impact of intermittent fasting on health and disease processes. *Ageing Research Reviews, 39*(1), 46–58. https://doi.org/10.1016/j.arr.2016.10.005

Mayo Clinic Staff. (2019). *How heart disease is different for women*. Mayo Clinic. https://www.mayoclinic.org/diseases-conditions/heart-disease/in-depth/heartdisease/art-20046167

Mayo Clinic Staff. (2022, November 2). *Low-glycemic index diet: What's behind the claims?* Mayo Clinic. https://www.mayoclinic.org/healthy-lifestyle/nutrition-and-healthy-eating/in-depth/low-glycemic-index-diet/art-20048478

Meimand, E. H. A., & Moghaddam, J. M. K. (2023). Evaluation of fasting effects during the Holy month of Ramadan on patients with epileptic attacks who visited the Emergency Room. *Journal of Kerman University of Medical Sciences, 30*(5), 267-270. doi:10.34172/jkmu.2023.45

Meule, A. (2020). The psychology of food cravings: The role of food deprivation. *Current Nutrition Reports, 9*(3), 251–257. https://doi.org/10.1007/s13668-020-00326-0

Mircica, I. (2022, December 1). *5 benefits of adopting intermittent fasting for seniors' health.* Morada Senior Living. https://www.moradaseniorliving.com/senior-living-blog/5-benefits-of-adopting-intermittent-fasting-for-seniors-health/

Mount Sinai. (2019, August 22). *Mount Sinai researchers discover that fasting reduces inflammation and improves chronic inflammatory diseases.* Mount Sinai Health System. https://www.mountsinai.org/about/newsroom/2019/mount-sinairesearchers-discover-that-fasting-reduces-inflammation-and-improves-chronic-inflammatory-diseases

Nazish, N. (2021, June 30). 10 intermittent fasting myths you should stop believing. *Forbes.* https://www.forbes.com/sites/nomanazish/2021/06/30/10-intermittent-fastingmyths-you-should-stop-believing

Neuroscience News. (2023, June 8). *Stressed brains amplify comfort food cravings.* https://neurosciencenews.com/stress-food-craving-23423/

NHS. (2018, June 26). *What is the glycaemic index (GI)?* https://www.nhs.uk/common-health-questions/food-and-diet/what-is-theglycaemic-index-gi/

Noguchi-Shinohara, M., Yuki, S., Dohmoto, C., Ikeda, Y., Samuraki, M., Iwasa, K., Yokogawa, M., Asai, K., Komai, K., Nakamura, Hl, & Yamada, M. (2014). Consumption of green tea, but not black tea or coffee, is associated with reduced risk of cognitive decline. *PloS one, 9*(5), e96013. https://doi.org/10.1371/journal.pone.0096013

Pacheco, D., & Singh, A. (2020, September 4). *Alcohol and sleep.* Sleep Foundation. https://www.sleepfoundation.org/nutrition/alcohol-and-sleep

Panoff, L. (2019, September 26). *What breaks a fast? Foods, drinks, and supplements.* Healthline. https://www.healthline.com/nutrition/what-breaks-a-fast

Parker, K. (2021, June 2). *The effect of intermittent fasting on your brain.* Aviv Clinics USA. https://aviv-clinics.com/blog/nutrition/the-effect-of-intermittent-fasting-on-your-brain/

Payne, K. (2023, May 12). *How writing can help you heal and transform.* New Thinking. https://www.newthinking.com/health/how-writing-can-help-youheal-and-transform

Payton, L. T. (2023, June 26). *Intermittent fasting versus calorie counting for weight loss:*

Many of the benefits are similar. Fortune Well. https://fortune.com/well/2023/06/26/intermittent-fasting-calorie-countingbenefits/

Pursuit. (2017, April 12). *The effect of vitamin B12 on carbohydrate and lipid metabolism*. Pursuit Training Center. https://pursuit.fit/nutritional-science/theeffect-of-vitamin-b12-on-carbohydrate-and-lipid-metabolism/

Phillips, M. C. L. (2019). Fasting as a therapy in neurological disease. *Nutrients, 11*(10). https://doi.org/10.3390/nu11102501

Quick fish salad with mackerel. (n.d.). Optimising Nutrition. https://optimisingnutrition.com/fish-and-salad-lunch/

Rath, L. (2022, December 26). *Get the latest news about rheumatoid arthritis & heart disease today!* Arthritis Foundation. https://www.arthritis.org/healthwellness/about-arthritis/related-conditions/other-diseases/rheumatoidarthritis-heart-disease

Richter, A., & Ajmera, R. (2018, July 30). *8 health benefits of fasting, backed by science*. Healthline. https://www.healthline.com/nutrition/fasting-benefits

Richter, A., Snyder, C. & Gunnars, K. (2022, February 23). *5 intermittent fasting methods, reviewed*. Healthline. https://www.healthline.com/nutrition/6-ways-to-do-intermittent-fasting

Rodgers, J. L., Jones, J., Bolleddu, S. I., Vanthenapalli, S., Rodgers, L. E., Shah, K., Karia, K., & Panguluri, S. K. (2019). Cardiovascular risks associated with gender and aging. *Journal of Cardiovascular Development and Disease, 6*(2), 19. https://doi.org/10.3390/jcdd6020019

Rosario, C. (2021, May 6). *What women over the age of 50 should know about coronary heart disease prevention*. Cardio Diagnostics. https://cardiodiagnosticsinc.com/what-women-over-the-age-of-50-should-know-about-coronary-heart-disease-prevention/

Rosenfield, R. L., & Ehrmann, D. A. (2016). The pathogenesis of polycystic ovary syndrome (PCOS): The hypothesis of PCOS as functional ovarian hyperandrogenism revisited. *Endocrine Reviews, 37*(5), 467–520. https://doi.org/10.1210/er.2015-1104

Royal Osteoporosis Society. (n.d.). *Osteoporosis: Exercises for back pain*. https://theros.org.uk/information-and-support/osteoporosis/living-withosteoporosis/exercise-and-physical-activity-for-osteoporosis/caring-for-yourback/exercises-for-back-pain-after-spinal-fractures/

Ryskamp, S. (2019, July 29). *Intermittent Fasting: Is it Right for You?* Michigan Medicine. https://www/michiganmedicine.org/health-lab/intermittent-fasting-is-it-right-you

SciTechDaily.com. (2022, August 29). *8 ways to curb cravings during intermittent fasting*. SciTechDaily. https://scitechdaily.com/8-ways-to-curb-cravings-during-intermittent-fasting/

Shah, M. (2022, August 2). *A comparison of intermittent fasting and other diets.* HealthifyMe. https://www.healthifyme.com/blog/intermittent-fasting-and-other-diets/

Singh, M. (2022). *Who shouldn't follow intermittent fasting?* NDTV. https://www.ndtv.com/health/who-shouldnt-follow-intermittent-fasting-3264060

Sovetkina, A., Nadir, R., Fung, J. N. M., Nadjarpour, A., & Beddoe, B. (2020). The physiological role of ghrelin in the regulation of energy and glucose homeostasis. *Cureus, 12*(5). https://doi.org/10.7759/cureus.7941

Tinsley, G., & Hill, A. (2022, June 14). *Eat stop eat review: Does it work for weight loss?* Healthline. https://www.healthline.com/nutrition/eat-stop-eat-review#basics

Trepanowski, J. F., Kroeger, C. M., Barnosky, A., Klempel, M. C., Bhutani, S., Hoddy, K. K., Gabel, K., Freels, S., Rigdon, J., Rood, J., Ravussin, E., & Varady, K. A. (2017). Effect of alternate-day fasting on weight loss, weight maintenance, and cardioprotection among metabolically healthy obese adults. *JAMA Internal Medicine, 177*(7), 930. https://doi.org/10.1001/jamainternmed.2017.0936

Varady, K. A. (2022). Effect of Intermittent Fasting on Reproductive Hormone Levels in Females and Males: A Review of Human Trials. *Nutrients, 14*(11), 2343. https://doi.org/10.3390/nu14112343

Wang, Y., & Wu, R. (2022). The effect of fasting on human metabolism and psychological health. *Disease Markers, 2022*, 1–7. https://doi.org/10.1155/2022/5653739

WebMD Editorial Contributors. (2021a, September 27). *What to know about intermittent fasting for women after 50.* WebMD. https://www.webmd.com/healthy-aging/what-to-know-about-intermittent-fasting-for-women-after-50

WebMD Editorial Contributors. (2021b, October 25). *Worst carbs for adults over 50.* WebMD. https://www.webmd.com/healthy-aging/worst-carbs-for-adults-over50

West, H. (2021, July 19). *Does intermittent fasting boost your metabolism?* Healthline. https://www.healthline.com/nutrition/intermittent-fastingmetabolism#metabolism-boost

Whitcomb, B. W., Purdue-Smithe, A. C., Szegda, K., L., Boutot, M. E., Hankinson, S. E., Manson, J. E., Rosner, B., Willett, W. C., Eliassen, A. H., & Bertone-Johnson, E. R. (2018). Cigarette smoking and risk of early natural menopause. *American Journal of Epidemiology, 187*(4), 696-704. https://doi.org/10.1093/aje/kwx292

World Health Organisation. (2022, October 17). *Menopause.* https://www.who.int/news-room/fact-sheets/detail/menopause

Yao, Z.-F., & Hsieh, S. (2019). Neurocognitive mechanism of human resilience: A conceptual framework and empirical review. *International Journal of*

Environmental Research and Public Health, 16(24), 5123. https://doi.org/10.3390/ijerph16245123

Yasuda, J., Tomita, T., Arimitsu, T., & Fujita, S. (2020). Evenly Distributed Protein Intake over 3 Meals Augments Resistance Exercise-Induced Muscle Hypertrophy in Healthy Young Men. *The Journal of nutrition, 150*(7), 1845–1851. https://doi.org/10.1093/jn/nxaa101

Yeung, A. Y., & Tadi, P. (2023). *Physiology, obesity neurohormonal appetite and satiety control.* National Library of Medicine. https://www.ncbi.nlm.nih.gov/books/NBK555906

Zietsman, G. (2020, September 29). Study recommends a combo of Mediterranean diet and intermittent fasting for the heart. *News24*. https://www.news24.com/life/archive/study-recommends-combo-of-mediterranean-diet-and-intermittent-fasting-for-the-heart-20200929-3

Zouhal, H., Saeidi, A., Salhi, A., Li, H., Essop, M. F., Laher, I., Rhibi, F., Amani Shalamzari, S., & Ben Abderrahman, A. (2020). Exercise training and fasting: Current insights. *Open Access Journal of Sports Medicine, Volume 11*(2), 1–28. https://doi.org/10.2147/oajsm.s224919

Image References

OpenAI. (2024). *ChatGPT* (4) [Large language model]. https://chat.openai.com
Lioputrahard. Depositphotos.com

Made in the USA
Las Vegas, NV
08 July 2024